READER'S DIGEST

FOODS
THAT
HARM
FOODS
THAT
HEAL

This special edition is adapted from
Foods That Harm, Foods That Heal
An A-Z Guide to Safe and Healthy Eating

NOTE TO READERS:

Information in this book should not be substituted for, or
used to alter, medical therapy without your doctor's advice.
For specific health problems, consult your physician.

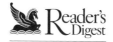

Reader's Digest

The Reader's Digest Association (Canada) Ltd., Montreal

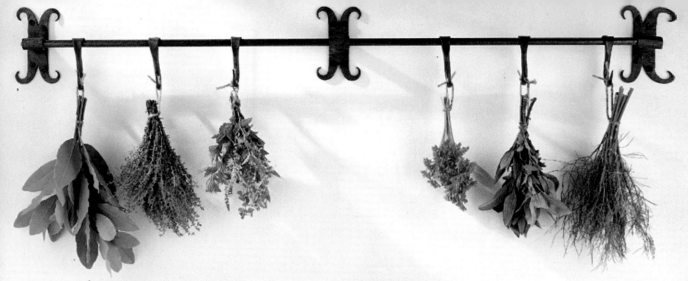

PROJECT EDITORS: **Anita Winterberg,
Suzanne E. Weiss**
PROJECT ART EDITOR: **Marisa Gentile Raffio**
DESIGNER: **Andrée Payette**
EDITOR: **Theresa Lane**
COPY EDITOR: **Gilles Humbert**
EDITORIAL ASSISTANT: **Vita Gardner**
SENIOR ASSOCIATE ART EDITOR: **Todd Victor**
ASSOCIATE ART EDITOR: **Bruce R. McKillip**
PICTURE RESEARCHER: **Rachel Irwin**

EDITORIAL ADMINISTRATOR: **Elizabeth Eastman**
PRODUCTION MANAGER: **Holger Lorenzen**
COORDINATOR: **Susan Wong**
CONSULTANT: **Joseph A. Schwarcz, Ph.D.**

READER'S DIGEST BOOKS AND
HOME ENTERTAINMENT
EDITORIAL DIRECTOR: **Deirdre Gilbert**
MANAGING EDITOR: **Philomena Rutherford**
ART DIRECTOR: **John McGuffie**

CONTRIBUTORS

EDITORIAL DIRECTOR/PRODUCER
Genell J. Subak-Sharpe, M.S.

MEDICAL CONSULTANTS
Morton D. Bogdonoff, M.D.
 Professor of Medicine
 New York Hospital–Cornell Medical Center
Karen Levine, R.D.
 Staff Dietitian
 Harlem Hospital Center

WRITERS/EDITORS
Arlyn Apollo
Diana Benzaia
Jean Callahan
Mikola De Roo
Nicole Freeland
Emily Paulsen
Rosemary Perkins
Ann Forer Stockton

RESEARCHERS
Helene MacLean
Sarah Subak-Sharpe

COPY EDITORS
Gina Grant
Diana Marsh
Joseph Marchetti
Judy Yelon

ILLUSTRATORS
Julia Bigg
Dick Bonson
Glynn Boyd Harte
Clare Melinsky
Francis Scappatricci
Lesli Sternberg
Sam Thompson
Charlotte Wess

PHOTOGRAPHERS
Karl Adamson
Colin Cooke
Gus Filgate
Vernon Morgan
Carol Sharpe
Jon Stewart

FOOD STYLISTS
Nir Adar
Karen Temple

For information on this and other Reader's Digest products, or to request a catalogue,
please call our 24-hour Customer Service hotline at 1-888-465-0780.
You can also visit us on the World Wide Web at http://www.readersdigest.ca

ISBN 0-88850-744-5

Printed in Canada   01 02 03 / 3 2 1

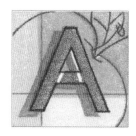

ACNE

EAT PLENTY OF
- *Fresh fruits and vegetables for vitamins A and C.*
- *Whole grains and cereals for B vitamins and zinc.*
- *Lean meat, poultry, and fish for zinc.*

AVOID
- *Kelp supplements.*
- *Iodized salt.*
- *High doses of B vitamins.*

Almost everyone experiences an occasional flare-up of acne—usually just a few blackheads and pimples, less often deep, scarring cysts. Although acne can occur at any age, it is most prevalent during adolescence, afflicting 85 percent of all teenagers to varying degrees.

Dermatologists stress that diet and other lifestyle factors, including cleanliness and sexual activity, do not cause acne. Still, parents and even some teen magazines keep the diet myth alive by insisting that eating chocolate, French fries, sweets, and other high-fat, sugary teen favorites can lead to acne. In rare instances, sensitivity to a food may exacerbate existing acne, but it is unlikely that any food actually causes it. (An exception is kelp, a seaweed sold as a dietary supplement or a salt substitute; it can cause severe cystic acne. Iodized salt can also provoke an acne flare-up.)

Hormones are responsible for most cases of acne. The surge of androgens (male sex hormones) that occurs during puberty prompts the skin's oil (sebaceous) glands to enlarge and increases the production of sebum, the oily substance that lubricates the skin. Boys are more severely affected by acne than girls. Still, even adult women find that acne flares up in periods of hormonal change, such as before menstruation, during pregnancy, or at the time of menopause.

Androgens also stimulate the growth of body hair and cause increased shedding of the cells that line follicles, the skin cavities from which hair grows. This cellular debris then clogs pores and blocks the flow of sebum; the resulting swollen glands form a whitehead, or closed comedo. If part of the pore remains open, the sebum exposed to oxygen darkens and becomes a blackhead; any inflammation will result in a pus-filled pimple. Cystic acne, the most severe form, develops when the blocked glands become infected by bacteria that normally inhabit the skin.

Because severe acne tends to run in families, heredity is suspected of playing a role in causing it. A number of medications can also cause acne; major offenders include steroids and other hormonal agents, iodine preparations, lithium, anticonvulsants, and drugs used to treat tuberculosis. The use of oily makeup can further clog pores and worsen acne; exposure to industrial oils and chemicals, such as naphthalenes and biphenyls, can cause acne too.

Stress often triggers a flare-up of acne, most likely by altering hormone levels. In turn, hormonal changes can stimulate food cravings, especially for chocolates and other sweets. Consequently, the acne sufferer may erroneously attribute the acne to gorging on chocolates or sweets, rather than stress, the real culprit for both.

DIET AND SKIN HEALTH

Clear, glowing skin reflects overall good health. This requires not only a balanced diet but also regular exercise, adequate sleep, and avoiding such detrimental habits as smoking and excessive exposure of the skin to sun. Vitamins A and C are essential for building and maintaining healthy skin; a daily diet that provides five or more servings of fresh vegetables and fruits (at least one citrus) will provide adequate amounts of these nutrients. B vitamins are thought to regulate sebum production; whole-grain cereals and breads, dried beans and other legumes, and lean meats are excellent sources of these vitamins. These foods also provide good amounts of zinc, a mineral that some studies link to skin health.

Some teenagers attempt to self-treat acne with high-dose vitamin and mineral supplements, an approach that can actually worsen the condition. Recent studies show that high doses of vitamins B_1, B_6, and B_{12} can trigger acne, and high doses of vitamin A can cause dry, flaking skin and hair loss.

ACNE TREATMENTS

Once or twice a day, gently wash the skin with a mild, nonmedicated unscented soap, rinse with cool water, and pat dry. Avoid scrubbing or using abrasive pads or grains—these irritate the skin and can even worsen acne. If the skin is very oily, wipe it gently with a cotton ball soaked in witch hazel. Use water-based, unscented cosmetics.

Most persistent mild to moderate acne can usually be controlled with nonprescription drugs, such as 2.5- or 5-percent strength benzoyl peroxide gel, lotion, or ointment. Start with a nightly application, and after a week add a morning application. Improvement should occur within 3 weeks; if not, try a stronger 10-percent solution.

A dermatologist may prescribe tretinoin, a topical medication derived from vitamin A; an antibiotic, in either topical or pill form, may also be tried. Isotretinoin (Accutane), a potent oral drug, is reserved for severe cystic acne.

ADDITIVES: HELPFUL OR HARMFUL?

For centuries, people have enhanced their foods with various flavorings, preservatives, and dyes. Still, consumers worry that some of the food additives in use today may be harmful.

Few foods reach today's supermarkets free of additives, substances that do not occur naturally in a food. These include preservatives to prevent spoilage; emulsifiers to prevent water and fat from separating; thickeners; vitamins and minerals, either to replace nutrients lost in processing or to increase nutritional value; sugar, artificial sweeteners, salt, and other flavorings to improve taste; and dyes to make everything from oranges to soft drinks more visually appealing.

In all, Canadian food processors may use any of about 2,800 additives. Although many people question the safety of these additives, there is little evidence that they constitute a major health risk for most people. In fact, thanks to some of these additives, Canadians enjoy history's safest and most abundant assortment of foods.

The most common food additives are sugar, corn syrup, other sweeteners, and salt; they are used both to enhance flavor and to retard spoilage. Many other additives offer their own unique health benefits; these include calcium, as well as ascorbic acid (vitamin C),

---

BENEFITS
- *Prevent spoilage and rancidity.*
- *Enhance flavor and appearance.*
- *Boost nutritional content.*

DRAWBACKS
- *Susceptible people may suffer allergic or adverse reactions.*
- *Some can exacerbate medical conditions.*

---

vitamin E, and other ANTIOXIDANTS that prevent fats from turning rancid and also may protect against cancer, heart disease, and other diseases.

More problematic, at least to the public, are substances with strange chemical names like sodium stearyl fumarate (an additive to improve the texture and handling properties of baked goods)

and dioctyl sodium sulfosuccinate (an emulsifier and flavor enhancer in processed foods). These substances are considered harmless, but consumers who don't understand why such chemical compounds are added to foods are understandably wary.

THE QUESTIONABLE FEW

The majority of food additives are without a doubt safe, but there are exceptions, and every now and then, one is removed from the market. The fact that some dyes, such as Red # 2, are allowed in Canada but are banned in the U.S. demonstrates that in some cases, "safety" is open to interpretation. On the other hand, controversial actions have

HIDDEN EXTRAS.
Accidental additives, such as pesticides and the hormones fed to some farm animals, make their way into our food.

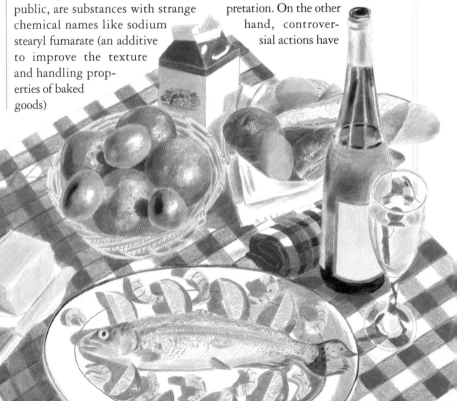

COMMON FOOD ADDITIVES

Consumer concerns over food additives often stem from misinformation or confusion over long chemical names.

All new additives receive federal government approval; older additives are presumed to be generally safe.

TYPE OF ADDITIVE	FOUND IN	FUNCTION
PRESERVATIVES		
Antimicrobials		
Benzoic acid and benzoates	Soft drinks, beer, fruit products, margarine, acidic foods.	Extend shelf life and protect food from fungi and bacteria.
Nitrites and nitrates	Processed meats, such as sausages, hot dogs, bacon, ham, and lunch meats. Smoked fish.	Extend shelf life and protect food from fungi and bacteria; preserve color in meats and dried fruits.
Sulfites	Dried fruits, shredded coconut, fruit-based pie fillings, relishes.	Extend shelf life and protect food from fungi and bacteria.
Antioxidants		
Ascorbic acid (vitamin C) and ascorbates	Fruit products (juices, jams, and canned fruits), acidic foods, and fatty foods that become rancid.	Ascorbates prevent fruit juices from turning brown and fatty foods from becoming rancid. They also improve baking quality in wheat.
BHA or BHT	Fatty foods that can turn rancid, such as baked products, cereals, potato chips, and fats and oils. 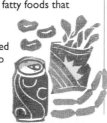	Prevents fatty foods from turning rancid when exposed to oxygen.
Tocopherols (vitamin E)	Oils and shortenings.	Prevent rancidity in fats and other damage to food due to exposure to oxygen.
COLORINGS		
Beta carotene	Many processed foods, especially sweets and products marketed for children, soft drinks, baked goods, and confectionery items, such as frosting, jams, and margarine. Also used in bologna and other processed meats as well as to color the skins of oranges and certain other fruits.	Make food look more appetizing by meeting people's food color expectations; for example, turning cherry Jell-O red.
Caramel		
Carrot oil		
Citrus red # 1		
Dehydrated beets		
FD&C colors: Blue # 1, 2; Red # 2; Yellow # 5, 6		
FLAVOR ENHANCERS		
Dioctyl sodium-sulfosuccinate	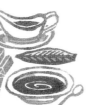 Mixes, processed foods.	Improve the flavor of many canned or processed foods.
Disodium guanylate	Canned meats, meat-based foods.	
Hydrolyzed vegetable protein	Mixes, stock, processed meats.	
Monosodium glutamate (MSG)	Chinese food, dry mixes, stock cubes, and canned, processed, and frozen meats.	Heightens taste perception so that foods seem to taste better.
EMULSIFIERS, STABILIZERS, AND THICKENERS		
Carrageenan	Sauces, soups, breads, baked goods, frozen desserts, ice cream, low-fat and artificial cream cheese, condiments, jams, jellies, chocolate, puddings, and milk shakes.	Improve texture and consistency of processed foods by increasing smoothness, creaminess, and volume. Hold in moisture and prevent separation of oil and water. Excessive pectin can result in bloating.
Cellulose		
Glycerol		
Guar gum		
Gum arabic		
Lecithin		
Pectins		

MONOSODIUM GLUTAMATE

Used as a flavor enhancer, monosodium glutamate (MSG) is a common ingredient in Oriental cooking. It tastes salty and slightly bitter, but does not actually change the flavor of food. Instead, it acts on the tongue to heighten the perception of certain tastes and minimize others. Thus, it masks the unpleasant taste of fermented or slightly spoiled foods and brings out other more agreeable flavors.

MSG occurs naturally in dried seaweed; more commonly, it is made from wheat or corn gluten or the liquid waste of sugar-beet refining. In susceptible people, MSG may trigger headaches, various idiosyncratic reactions, or a flare-up of celiac disease symptoms.

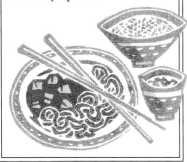

fueled worries about complete groups of additives in some instances. The case of artificial sweeteners is a prime example. Cyclamates were banned in the U.S. in 1969, when a group of researchers reported an apparent increased incidence of cancer in rats fed large amounts of the sweetener. Canadian authorities were not convinced that this study showed a risk for humans, and Canada, and at least 40 other countries, allows the use of cyclamates. Saccharin, on the other hand, is allowed as an additive in the U.S.; in Canada, however, it may be sold only as a tabletop sweetener. The issue, once again, is possible carcinogenicity based on studies of rats fed massive amounts of saccharin, but humans have been using saccharin for over a hundred years with no ill effects. Aspartame was approved despite concerns over its potential problems for people with phenylketonuria, a rare hereditary metabolic disorder. Some studies also suggest that in isolated cases aspartame can trigger seizures or headaches, but the vast majority use it without obvious problems.

ACCIDENTAL ADDITIVES

Some 10,000 substances make their way into food during growing, processing, and packaging; some of these accidental additives can pose more of a health threat than preservatives and other direct additives. Some foods, for example, contain traces of pesticides sprayed on crops or applied to the soil. Environmental pollutants in foods, such as PCBs, mercury, and lead, are harmful when ingested in large quantities.

Sometimes allergic reactions that are blamed on foods or intentional additives are actually triggered by an unintended additive. For example, a person who has never had a food allergy may inexplicably develop hives or a rash after drinking milk. In some cases, allergists have traced the symptoms to penicillin rather than to the milk itself. How does this antibiotic get into milk? Mastitis, a common problem in cows, is treated with penicillin injected directly into the udder. The resulting small amounts of penicillin in the milk would not be harmful for most people, only to those who are allergic to the drug.

A PRUDENT APPROACH

Even though the benefits of most food additives outweigh any potential risks, prudence and moderation should prevail in their use, and some can be avoided entirely. A person concerned about food dyes, for example, usually can buy natural items, such as undyed oranges, which may have a mottled, pale yellow or green-tinged skin. The natural fruit may not be as pretty as the color-treated, but it will taste as good or perhaps even better, because it has ripened longer on the tree.

Some additives pose problems for people with certain medical conditions. Anyone with high blood pressure or any condition that mandates a low-salt diet should check the labels on all processed foods for various forms of sodium, all of which contain salt. Similarly, people trying to reduce sugar intake should look for lactose and other ingredients ending in "ose"; these are forms of sugar. Those with an inherited tendency to store excessive iron, a condition called hemochromatosis, should avoid iron-enriched breads, cereals, and other products. Sulfites used to preserve the color of dried fruits, frozen French fries, and sauerkraut can trigger an asthma attack in susceptible people.

Some additives amount to overkill; this is especially true of highly fortified cereals. It's unrealistic to expect a bowl of cereal to provide 100 percent of the Recommended Nutrient Intake (RNI) for a dozen or more vitamins and minerals; a high-fiber, whole-grain cereal is just as healthful. Calcium is now added to orange juice, bread, and a variety of other foods. These products may be fine for someone who shuns milk and other foods naturally high in calcium, but may actually be harmful to people who suffer from rare conditions such as milk-alkali syndrome, characterized by too much calcium in the blood.

Remember, too, that preserved foods have more additives than their fresh counterparts. Fresh meat, poultry, and fish do not contain the nitrates and other preservatives found in smoked or processed meats.

AGING AND DIET

As you get older, your body's energy needs drop; at the same time, demands for some nutrients increase. New studies indicate some of these can slow the aging process.

While aging is inevitable, many of the degenerative changes that prevail among the elderly are not if preventive steps are taken. Recent medical research confirms that good nutrition can prevent or at least slow such debilitating conditions as osteoporosis, diabetes, and heart disease. In fact, one report estimates that one-third to one-half of the health problems of people over the age of 65 are related to diet. In contrast, various studies of Mormons, Seventh-Day Adventists, and Trappist monks—all people who follow a vegetarian diet and engage in a prudent lifestyle—show that they enjoy increased life expectancy.

On the whole, the elderly are the most poorly nourished group of all North Americans. There are many reasons for this: A person's appetite and the senses of taste and smell decline with age, making food considerably less appealing. Many older people experience difficulty chewing; in addition, heartburn, constipation, lactose intolerance, and other digestive problems increase with age and contribute to poor nutrition. The loss of a partner, or difficulty in shopping or preparing meals, may result in a person subsisting on tea, toast, sweets, canned soups, and other convenience foods that provide little nutrition.

A number of older people living on a fixed income usually cannot afford such nutritious foods as fresh fruits, vegetables, fish, and meat. Also, some of them fall victim to nutrition quackery or engage in misguided self-treatment with high-dose vitamins and minerals. None of these problems are insoluble, but finding solutions to them may take a bit of effort (see Practical Tips, p.9).

CHANGING NEEDS

A person's body composition changes with age, as muscle mass decreases, often due to disuse, and fatty tissue increases. Because metabolism slows down, fewer calories are required; experts estimate that the average person should consume 10 percent fewer calories for every decade after the age of 50. Therefore, a 50-year-old who needs 1,800 calories a day will require 1,440 at age 70, and perhaps even fewer if he is sedentary. People who

AN APPETITE FOR LIVING. *A meal is always more enjoyable when shared with friends. Try to eat a balanced diet, whatever your age.*

BASIC DIETARY RECOMMENDATIONS

The National Institute on Aging in the United States recommends that an older person's daily diet include the minimum number of servings outlined below. Sugar, salt, and fats should be used sparingly; alcohol should be consumed only in moderation, defined as one drink a day for women and two for men.

FOOD GROUP	PROVIDES
STARCHES (COMPLEX CARBOHYDRATES)	
At least 5 servings: Whole grains, breads, and cereals; brown rice, kasha, millet, and other grains; dried beans, peas, lentils, and other legumes; potatoes, pasta, and other starchy foods.	Thiamine, riboflavin, niacin, folate, B_6 and other B vitamins; fiber; and complete protein when grains and legumes are combined.
VEGETABLES AND FRUITS	
At least 5 servings: Fresh vegetables and fruits, including dark green leafy vegetables, such as broccoli, cabbage, kale, and spinach; yellow vegetables, such as carrots and squash; citrus fruits, berries, tomatoes, bananas, and other fruits.	Vitamins C and A, beta carotene, riboflavin, folate, various minerals, and fiber. These are needed to prevent deficiency disorders and may protect against cancer.
HIGH-PROTEIN FOODS	
At least 2 servings: Lean beef, lamb, chicken and other poultry; fish and other seafood; eggs, tofu, and a combination of grains and legumes.	Thiamine, riboflavin, niacin, and vitamins E, B_6, and B_{12}; iron, zinc, and other minerals. Canned sardines and salmon with bones provide calcium.
DAIRY PRODUCTS	
At least 2 servings: Low-fat milk, cheese, yogurt, and other milk products. (Choose lactose-reduced milk and yogurt if you have trouble digesting regular milk.)	Protein, calcium, vitamins A and D. Needed to prevent the loss of bone minerals that frequently occurs with increasing age.

fail to cut back on food intake are likely to gain weight, increasing the risk of heart disease, diabetes, and osteoarthritis.

With increasing age, the body is less efficient in absorbing and using some nutrients; osteoporosis and other medical conditions common among older people also change nutritional needs. Consequently, an older person is likely to need extra amounts of the following essential nutrients:

Calcium to prevent osteoporosis and maintain healthy bones.

Vitamin D, which the body needs in order to absorb the calcium.

Vitamin B_{12} to build red blood cells and maintain healthy nerves.

Vitamin E to help protect against heart disease.

Zinc to help compensate for lowered immunity due to aging.

Potassium, especially in the presence of high blood pressure or the use of diuretic drugs.

Fiber to prevent constipation.

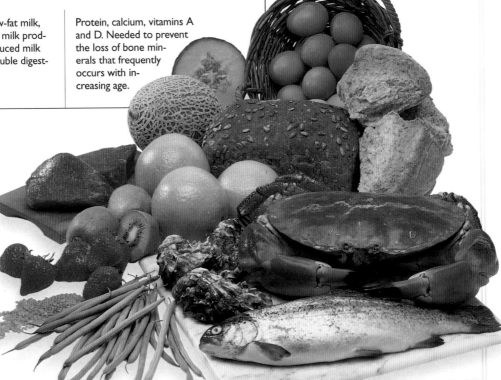

A LITTLE VARIETY. A balanced diet that contains a wide assortment of fresh foods will usually provide all the vitamins, minerals, and energy that an older person needs to maintain optimal health and vitality.

Some doctors recommend a daily vitamin and mineral supplement to ensure that an older person takes in 100 percent of the Recommended Nutrient Intakes (RNIs). Others feel this is unnecessary if the person eats a varied diet (see Basic Dietary Recommendations, facing page). In any event, high-dose supplements should be avoided unless recommended by a physician or dietitian, as they can lead to nutritional imbalances. For example, zinc supplements can interfere with the body's use of folic acid; iron can inhibit proper calcium and zinc absorption; vitamin A overdose can even cause death.

PRACTICAL TIPS

• Plan meals for regular times during the day rather than snacking.
• Strive to make meals pleasurable, even if you're eating alone. Set the table or prepare an attractive tray. Turn on your favorite music to improve your mood.
• If you dislike eating alone, organize regular potluck meals with friends and neighbors. Or consider joining an organization that provides an opportunity to dine with others.
• Select foods that provide contrasts in color, texture, and flavor. Avoid adding salt to improve flavor; instead, use herbs and spices. A sprinkling of nutmeg or cinnamon can compensate for a diminished sense of taste.
• A small glass of wine or beer with a meal aids digestion and adds to eating pleasure. But don't substitute alcohol for food, and check with your doctor to make sure that it does not interact with any medications you might be taking.
• Make sure you drink six to eight glasses of water, juice, or other nonalcoholic fluid a day. Older people often experience decreased thirst or they reduce fluid intake because of bladder-control problems. This can contribute to constipation and kidney problems

Case Study

Joe, a 71-year-old retired accountant, had never paid much attention to shopping and cooking—his wife had always taken care of those chores. When his wife died, Joe found mealtimes increasingly trying. He didn't like to eat alone in restaurants, although now and then he'd go on an excursion to pick up a sandwich from the neighborhood deli. Joe tried frozen TV dinners a few times but rarely enjoyed the way they tasted. About the only time he had a real meal was when friends invited him to eat with them. Otherwise, Joe's diet consisted of cold cereal and canned beans or soup.

Over several months, Joe came down with a number of colds. He often felt tired and listless, feelings that he attributed to lingering sadness and loneliness after his wife's death.

When Joe's sister, Elsa, came to visit for a few days, she was appalled by his diet and emotional state. "You're not getting any vegetables or fruits," she admonished him. "No wonder you feel run-down and catch one cold after another!" Still, she realized that nagging would not

get Joe out of his doldrums; he needed motivation and guidance.

Elsa found that the local Seniors Center had a daily lunch program; even better, she learned the center also offered a cooking course. Elsa finally convinced Joe to check out the latter.

Happily, the cooking class turned out to be exactly what Joe needed. He enjoyed learning to make interesting meals, and a trip to the supermarket gave Joe insight into buying fresh produce. Some fellow students were also without partners, and they began to cook and eat together.

At the urging of the class instructor, Joe helped organize weekly home cooking sessions, in which class members took turns playing host. Between sessions, Joe practiced his new food shopping and preparation skills. As he later confided to his sister, the cooking classes helped change his life. Joe not only found new friends and an enjoyable hobby, but he also began to pay more attention to eating a balanced, healthful diet.

and increase the risk of dehydration in hot weather.
• If you have trouble chewing, there's no need to resort to a bland liquid diet, which can lead to constipation and perhaps even malnutrition. Instead, prepare fish or ground meat and purée vegetables, soups, and other nutritious foods.
• Take daily walks or engage in other

exercise, but first consult your doctor for an appropriate routine. Exercise not only preserves muscle strength but also improves appetite and mood.
• If you're on a tight budget, organize a shopping co-op with others in a similar situation. Buying larger quantities is more economical; share with others, or divide the food into smaller portions and freeze them for future use.

AIDS AND HIV INFECTION

CONSUME PLENTY OF

- *Meat, liver, eggs, milk, and other high-calorie, high-protein foods to prevent weight and muscle loss.*
- *Pasta and other starchy foods, cooked vegetables, pasteurized juices, and canned or stewed fruits for essential vitamins and minerals.*

CUT DOWN ON

- *Fatty foods and whole-grain products if they cause diarrhea.*
- *Coffee, tea, and other caffeinated drinks that can cause diarrhea and reduce absorption of some nutrients.*

AVOID

- *Raw or undercooked foods, especially shellfish, eggs, and rare or uncooked processed meats.*
- *Alcohol, which can worsen diarrhea and interact with AIDS medications.*

There is still no cure for AIDS (acquired immune deficiency syndrome), nor is there a special diet for people infected with HIV, the human immunodeficiency virus that causes the disease. But good nutrition can help prevent or delay weight loss and other AIDS complications. Doctors often advise HIV-positive patients to consult a qualified clinical dietitian, preferably while still healthy, to learn about sound nutrition.

Asymptomatic HIV-infected individuals should follow the same dietary practices recommended for healthy people, but with added precautions. Because the HIV organism attacks the immune system, it makes a person more vulnerable to infections, including food poisoning from salmonella, shigella, campylobacter, and other bacteria. Such food-borne infections occur more frequently and are more severe in people with reduced immunity.

AIDS is a wasting disease, and death is often due to starvation rather than to other HIV complications. An AIDS patient should eat as much as possible and, unless markedly obese, not worry about gaining a few pounds. The extra weight can be critical in seeing a patient through a crisis when he can't eat.

Unfortunately, maintaining good nutrition is complicated by the ways in which AIDS affects the digestive system. It reduces absorption of nutrients, especially folate, riboflavin, thiamine, and vitamins B_6 and B_{12}; it often causes intractable diarrhea, which causes further nutritional loss; and it increases the risk of intestinal infections. Many AIDS patients also suffer appetite loss and bouts of nausea, either from the disease or from medications.

If rapid weight loss occurs, the patient may require artificial (hyperalimentation) feeding; this is generally administered through a gastric feeding tube inserted into the stomach or an intravenous line that pumps predigested nutrients into the bloodstream. Some AIDS specialists advise starting artificial feeding even before there is rapid weight loss, especially if nutrients are not being absorbed properly.

FOOD SAFETY

Anyone who is HIV-positive, or a person who prepares food for an AIDS patient, must pay special attention to food safety. Eggs should be boiled for at least 7 minutes or cooked until hard; meat and fish should be cooked until well done, with an internal temperature of 165°F (74°C) to 212°F (100°C). Raw oysters and other shellfish, sushi, steak tartare, rare hamburgers and roast beef as well as homemade mayonnaise and ice cream made with raw eggs must be avoided. Commercial mayonnaise and hard ice cream and sherbet are safe.

Fruits and vegetables are not as likely to cause problems as animal products. Even so, they should be washed carefully in soapy water and rinsed thoroughly. Many doctors advise following the same precautions as when traveling abroad; eat only cooked vegetables, and eat fruits that are peeled, stewed, or canned. Others feel that salads and some raw fruits and vegetables are safe but warn that these may be difficult for an AIDS patient to digest.

USE OF SUPPLEMENTS

Nutritionists generally recommend that HIV-positive people take a multiple vitamin and mineral pill to prevent nutritional deficiencies; however, supplements with more than 100 percent of the Recommended Nutrient Intakes (RNIs) should be used only if prescribed by a doctor. Many patients self-treat with high-dose supplements, a course that can lead to serious problems. High doses of vitamin C, for example, can worsen diarrhea.

Some self-help groups advocate taking high doses of zinc and selenium to bolster the immune system. There is no proof that supplements of these nutrients protect against AIDS-related infections; in fact, studies show that taking 200mg to 300mg of zinc a day for 6 weeks actually lowers immunity. Excessive selenium can also cause nausea, vomiting, and diarrhea.

Another dangerous dietary approach entails following a macrobiotic regimen, especially one that is restricted to brown rice and a few vegetables. Such a diet can actually worsen AIDS, because it fails to provide adequate nutrition; additionally, the excessive fiber can exacerbate diarrhea.

Herbal medicine is a popular self-care approach, though there is no evidence for its efficacy. Caution is needed as some herbal preparations contain substances that can cause serious side effects or interact with medications. Check with a doctor before taking any herbal or other preparation or engaging in self-treatment or alternative medicine.

ALCOHOL

BENEFITS
• *Moderate consumption cuts heart-attack risk by raising HDL cholesterol.*
• *In small amounts, it can improve appetite and aid digestion.*
• *May foster a happy mood.*

DRAWBACKS
• *Can provoke mood swings, aggression, and hangovers.*
• *Interacts with many medications.*
• *Over time, moderate to high intake increases the risk of cancers, stroke, heart and liver disease, and dementia.*

People have used alcohol in one form or another since prehistoric times. While alcohol is drunk for its mood-altering effects, in the past it was also used as an anesthetic, tonic, and disinfectant. Even today, alcohol is an ingredient in many over-the-counter medications.

Ethyl alcohol (ethanol), the main active ingredient of alcoholic beverages, is made by yeast fermentation of starch or sugar. Almost any sweet or starchy food—potatoes, grains, honey, grapes and other fruits, even dandelions—can be turned into alcohol.

Unlike most foods, alcohol is not digested; instead, 95 percent of it is absorbed into the bloodstream from the stomach and small intestine within an hour after ingestion. (The other 5 percent is eliminated through the kidneys, lungs, or skin.) The liver breaks down, or metabolizes, alcohol; the time this takes depends upon whether the alcohol is ingested with food and upon the person's sex, weight, body type, and tolerance level, which increases with time and use. On average, however, it takes the liver 3 to 5 hours to completely metabolize an ounce of alcohol.

Although the effect is the same over time, distilled liquors, such as whiskey and gin, have a more immediate impact than wines or beers, and all alcohol is

WHAT'S IN A DRINK

Alcohol contains 7 calories per gram, compared with 4 calories per gram of protein or carbohydrate and 9 calories per gram of fat. Some wines provide small amounts of iron and potassium, and beer contains niacin, vitamin B$_6$, chromium, and phosphorus. To benefit from the nutrients in these beverages, you would have to consume much more than the recommended limit of two drinks per day for a man or one for a woman. Each beverage listed below provides about ½ ounce of ethanol, the usual definition of a drink.

ITEM	ALCOHOL VOLUME	SERVING SIZE (OZ)	CALORIES
MIXED DRINKS WITH DISTILLED SPIRITS			
Bloody Mary	12%	5	116
Daiquiri	28%	2	111
Gin and tonic	9%	7.5	171
Manhattan	37%	2	128
Martini	38%	2.5	156
Piña colada	12%	4.5	262
Screwdriver	8%	7	174
Tequila sunrise	14%	5.5	189
Tom Collins	9%	7.5	121
Whiskey sour (using bottled mix)	17%	3.5	160
WINE AND WINE-RELATED PRODUCTS			
Regular wines	10%–14%	4	85
Sweet white wine	10%–14%	4	100
Light wines	6%–10%	5	65
Wine coolers (fruit juice, carbonated water, white wine, sugar)	3.5%–6%	12	220
Port	19%	4	158
Sherry	19%	3	125
ORDINARY BEER			
Regular	3%–5%	12	150
Light	3%–5%	12	100
STRONGER BREWED BEVERAGES			
Ales, porters, stouts, and malt liquors	5%–8%	12	150

COMPARISON OF UNIT MEASURES

½ oz ethanol = 1½ oz of 80-proof liquor = 4 oz or 5 oz of wine = 12 oz of beer absorbed more quickly when mixed with a carbonated beverage, such as club soda. Once in the bloodstream, alcohol reaches the brain in minutes. At first it acts as a stimulant, producing euphoria. This soon gives way to central nervous system depression and feelings of numbness, and finally to sleep or unconsciousness. Rapid ingestion of a large amount of alcohol can be fatal.

The term *proof* indicates alcohol concentrations; in Canada, proof is twice the alcohol content. Thus, a 90-proof liquor is 45 percent alcohol.

ALCOHOL AND CHOLESTEROL

Studies have found that drinking small amounts of alcohol, especially red wine, lowers the risk of a heart attack, presumably by reducing the detrimental effects of elevated blood cholesterol and by preventing clot formation. The mechanisms are unclear, but some researchers note that red wines contain BIOFLAVONOIDS (as do white wines in smaller amounts), a type of antioxidant. These substances protect cells from the damage that normally occurs when the body uses oxygen; they may also fortify LDL (low-density lipoprotein) cholesterol against oxidation (it's believed that oxidation of LDLs causes coronary arteries and other blood vessels to clog).

Other studies show that one or two drinks a day (see What's in a Drink, p.11) may increase the levels of protective HDL (high-density lipoprotein) cholesterol. But doctors note that even this amount of alcohol raises the risk of high blood pressure, stroke, liver disease, and certain cancers. They also suggest safer options; eating grapes, for example, provides even more bioflavonoids than wine, and aspirin is more effective in preventing clots.

ALCOHOL'S ADVERSE EFFECTS

Overconsumption of alcohol invariably results in a hangover; just how much is necessary to produce that misery de-

---

DID YOU KNOW?

• The hops that give beer its somewhat distinctive bitterness and aroma come from a vine that is a relative of cannabis.

• A cold shower, strong coffee, and similar folk remedies are of no value in helping a person sober up.

• Large amounts of alcohol lower sexual performance in men. Alcohol reduces levels of testosterone, the male sex hormone, while increasing estrogen levels, which can lead to impotence, shrunken testicles, and male breast growth.

---

pends on the biochemical individuality of the consumer, and the type of drink consumed. Symptoms may include thirst, headache, diarrhea, gastrointestinal upset, nausea, and irritability. Because of alcohol's diuretic effect, a person is likely to wake up feeling dehydrated; drinking water before going to bed may reduce these effects. The severity of a hangover is partially influenced by congeners, by-products of the fermentation process that contribute to the taste and aroma of an alcoholic beverage. The more congeners in a drink, the more severe a hangover may be. Brandy has the greatest number of congeners, followed by red wine, rum, whiskey, white wine, gin, and vodka.

Other, more serious effects of alcohol include the following:

Brain and nerves. Alcohol reduces blood flow to the brain and is also toxic to brain cells. Long-term overindulgence results in memory loss, nerve damage, and even dementia.

Liver. Because this organ metabolizes alcohol, it is vulnerable to damage, including a fatty liver, alcoholic hepatitis, and eventually scarring, or cirrhosis.

Heart. Even small amounts of alcohol may provoke cardiac arrhythmias. Long-term use of alcohol increases the risk of high blood pressure and heart

---

disease, especially cardiomyopathy, an enlargement and weakening of the heart muscle.

Digestive system. Alcohol raises the stomach's output of hydrochloric acid, which can worsen an ulcer. It also relaxes the sphincter between the esophagus and the stomach, resulting in heartburn from a backflow of acid.

EFFECTS ON NUTRITION

Small amounts of alcohol can stimulate appetite and aid digestion; overindulgence quickly erases the benefits. Even a weekend of heavy drinking causes a buildup of fatty cells in the liver. While this organ has remarkable recuperative powers, continued use can lead to permanent liver damage and problems in metabolizing glucose and various vitamins and minerals. These nutritional deficiencies can lead to other more serious conditions, such as anemia, nerve damage, and mental problems.

Long-term alcohol use often results in excessive weight gain, even though the person may consume less food. This is because alcohol is high in calories (see What's in a Drink, p.11) and is often consumed with fatty, high-calorie foods like salted peanuts and potato chips.

ALCOHOLISM

EAT PLENTY OF
• *Seafood, lean pork, and enriched cereals and breads for extra thiamine.*
• *Dark green leafy vegetables, oranges and other fresh fruits, poultry, and enriched cereals and breads for folate.*
• *Legumes, pasta, and other starchy foods for carbohydrate.*

AVOID
• *Alcohol in any form.*

In general, alcoholism is defined as chronic drinking that interferes with one's personal, family, or professional life. While an occasional drink is not likely to be harmful, it's important to recognize that alcohol is easily abused.

Factors that are thought to foster alcoholism include a genetic predisposition, learned behavior, and childhood experiences, including abuse. Progression of the disease varies from one person to another. For some, it develops as soon as they begin to drink; for most people, however, it progresses slowly from periodic social drinking to more frequent indulgence until finally the person is addicted.

Some alcoholics are binge drinkers and can go for weeks or even months without alcohol. But once they have a drink, they are unable to stop until they are incapacitated or pass out. Although these drinkers have difficulty maintaining sobriety, they are unlikely to suffer severe withdrawal symptoms when they abstain. In other cases, abstinence of 12 to 24 hours will produce withdrawal symptoms, such as sweating, irritability, nausea, vomiting, and weakness. More severe symptoms develop in 2 to 4 days and may include delirium tremens (DTs), a condition marked by fever and delirium.

EFFECTS OF ALCOHOLISM

Chronic overuse of alcohol takes a heavy psychological and physical toll. Alcoholics often do not appear to be intoxicated, but their ability to work and go about daily activities becomes increasingly impaired. They are very susceptible to depression, mood changes, and even violent behavior. Their suicide rate is higher than that of the general population. Alcoholics tend to be heavy smokers and may misuse other drugs, such as tranquilizers. On average, alcoholism shortens life expectancy, not only from suicide but also because it

HIGH AND LOW SPIRITS. *While alcohol can lift the spirits, too much can lead to depression and even aggression.*

raises the risk of other life-threatening diseases, including cancer of the pancreas, liver, and esophagus. Women who drink heavily while pregnant may have a baby with fetal alcohol syndrome, a constellation of birth defects, including mental retardation.

NUTRITIONAL EFFECTS

Alcoholism can lead to malnutrition, not only because chronic drinkers tend to have poor diets, but also because alcohol alters digestion and metabolism of most nutrients. Severe thiamine deficiency (marked by muscle cramps and wasting, nausea, appetite loss, nerve disorders, and depression) is extremely common, as are deficiencies of folate, riboflavin, vitamin B_6, and selenium. Disturbance of vitamin A metabolism can result in night blindness. Because many alcoholics suffer deficiency of vitamin D, which metabolizes calcium, they are at risk of bone fractures and osteoporosis. Impaired liver and pancreatic function may result in faulty fat digestion.

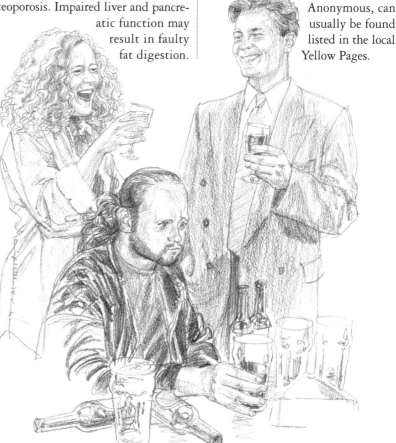

Since alcohol stimulates insulin production, glucose metabolism speeds up and can result in low blood sugar. In addition, alcoholics are often overweight, due to the calories in alcohol.

Once an alcoholic stops drinking, the nutritional problems are tackled one by one. Supplements are prescribed to treat deficiencies. A diet addresses underlying problems; for example, an overweight person needs a diet that reverses nutritional deficiencies without additional weight gain. If there is liver damage, protein intake must be monitored to prevent further liver problems.

MAINTAINING SOBRIETY

Abstinence, the only real treatment for alcoholism, is difficult to achieve and maintain. Withdrawal may require medical supervision and a stay in a hospital or clinic setting. Afterwards, support groups are critical. These groups, such as Alcoholics Anonymous, can usually be found listed in the local Yellow Pages.

ALLERGIC REACTIONS TO FOODS

*Scores of the ordinarily harmless substances in foods,
the air, and objects we touch can provoke symptoms ranging
from a runny nose and hives to fatal anaphylaxis.*

Allergies occur when our immune system overreacts to minute amounts of foreign substances. Approximately one in four North Americans—or some 70 million people—suffer from allergies. Of these, food allergies make up only a small percentage. Far more common are allergic reactions to pollen and other inhaled substances, medications, and substances that are absorbed into the skin.

Doctors do not completely understand why so many people have allergies, though heredity is instrumental. If both parents have allergies, their children will almost always follow suit, although the symptoms and allergens may be quite different. Food allergies in infants and children, however, tend to lessen as they grow, and the problem may disappear by adulthood.

Allergies basically develop in stages. When the immune system first encounters an allergen (or antigen)—a substance that it mistakenly perceives as a harmful foreign invader—it signals specialized cells to manufacture antibodies, or immunoglobulins, against it. The person will not experience an allergic reaction in that initial exposure; however, if the substance again enters the body, the antibodies programmed to mount an attack against it will go into action. In some instances, the response will not produce symptoms; but the stage will have been set. At some future date, an antigen-antibody reaction may provoke cells in the immune system to release large amounts of histamines and other chemicals that are responsible for an allergic response. When this happens, symptoms can range from something as mild as a sneeze or runny nose to an extremely serious reaction, such as sudden death.

COMMON SYMPTOMS

The most common symptoms of food allergies are nausea, vomiting, diarrhea, constipation, indigestion, headaches, skin rashes or hives, itching, shortness of breath (including asthma attacks), and, in severe cases, widespread swelling of the skin and mucous membranes. Swelling in the mouth or throat is potentially fatal because it can block the airways to the lungs. In the most severe cases, anaphylactic shock—a life-threatening collapse of the respiratory and circulatory system—may develop.

The allergen usually provokes the same symptoms each time, but many factors affect their intensity, including stress, how much of the offending food was eaten, how it was prepared, and whether it was eaten with other foods. Some people can tolerate small amounts of an offending food; others are so hypersensitive that they react to even a minute trace.

Most allergic reactions arise quickly, usually within a few minutes or up

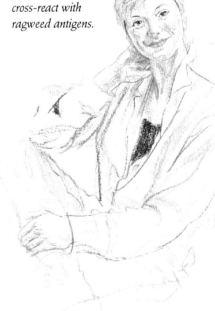

Case Study

Sharon, a 27-year-old teacher, suffered from hay fever during the ragweed season, but she was free of food allergies. One day a friend served her some chamomile tea; almost immediately, Sharon developed an itchy rash and swollen face.

Her friend, a nurse, suspected a severe allergic reaction and took her to the emergency room. Later tests confirmed that the chamomile tea had triggered Sharon's allergic response; she also reacted to related foods like artichokes, which have allergens that can cross-react with ragweed antigens.

to 2 hours after the allergen enters the body. In unusual cases, however, the reaction may be delayed for up to 48 hours, making it more difficult to identify the allergen.

PINPOINTING ALLERGENS

Some allergens are easily identified because characteristic symptoms will develop immediately after eating the offending food. In other instances, it may be necessary to keep a carefully documented diary of the time and content of all meals and snacks and the appearance and timing of any subsequent symptoms. After a week or two, a pattern may emerge. If so, eliminate the suspected food from the diet for at least a week, and then try it again. If symptoms develop only in the latter part of this experiment, chances are you have identified the offending food.

In more complicated cases, allergy tests may be required. The most common are skin tests; food extracts are placed on the skin, which is then scratched or pricked, allowing the penetration of a small amount of the extract. Development of a hive or itchy swelling usually indicates an allergic response. In some cases, a doctor may order a RAST (radioallergosorbent test) blood study in which small amounts of the patient's blood are mixed with food extracts and then analyzed for signs of antibody action. This test is more expensive than skin tests but may be safer for hypersensitive people, who may have a severe reaction to the skin test.

Still other tests may involve a medically supervised elimination diet and challenge tests. In one variation, the patient is put on a hypoallergenic diet of foods that are unlikely to cause allergies—for example, lamb, rice, carrots, sweet potatoes, and pears—for 7 to 10 days, at which time all allergic symptoms should completely disappear. (If they don't, a reaction to something other than food should be

COMMON FOOD ALLERGENS AND THEIR SYMPTOMS

Almost any food can provoke an allergic reaction. The following, listed in descending order with the most likely to occur at top, are the most common.

FOOD TYPES	PROBLEM FOODS	SYMPTOMS
Milk and milk products	Dairy products, such as milk, cheeses, yogurt, cream, ice cream, cream soups, and certain baked goods and desserts.	Constipation, diarrhea, and vomiting are most common; less frequent are rashes, hives, and breathing problems.
Eggs (especially egg whites)	Cakes, mousses, ice cream, sherbets, and other desserts; mayonnaise, salad dressings, French toast, waffles, and pancakes.	Rashes or hives, swelling, and intestinal upsets. Can trigger asthma attacks and eczema in some people.
Fish	Fresh, canned, smoked or pickled fish, fish-liver oils, caviar, foods containing fish, such as bisques, broths, and stews.	Rashes or hives, and perhaps red itchy eyes or a runny nose. Can trigger asthma attacks, diarrhea, and, rarely, anaphylaxis.
Shellfish	Crustaceans, such as shrimp, crab, lobster, and crayfish; mollusks, such as clams, oysters, and scallops; and seafood dishes.	Nausea, prolonged intestinal upsets, migraines, skin rashes, and swelling; possible anaphylaxis.
Wheat and wheat products	Cereals, bread or bread-related products, dry soup mixes, cakes, pasta, gravies, dumplings, products containing flour; beer and ale.	Diarrhea and other intestinal upsets, migraine headaches, and eczema.
Corn	Foods with corn as a vegetable, such as vegetable soup; baby foods (with cornstarch), baking mixes, processed meats, corn oils, margarine, salad dressings, MSG, and baked goods.	Rashes or hives, breathing problems, diarrhea and other intestinal upsets.
Nuts and peanuts	Candy and baked goods with pecans, walnuts, almonds, cashews, hazelnuts, pistachios, and peanuts; oils from nuts.	Intestinal upsets and breathing problems; possible anaphylaxis, usually when nuts are a hidden ingredient.
Fruits	Citrus fruits; in pollen-allergic persons, usually melons and other fruits with seeds.	Facial rash or hives, and itching or tingling sensations in the mouth.
Chocolate	Candy bars, baked goods, and other products containing cocoa or chocolate. (Testing often shows allergies are due to milk, nuts, or other ingredients added to chocolate.)	Rashes or hives; if milk or nuts are the real culprit, reactions may be more severe.

15

suspected.) The doctor then administers small amounts of food or food extracts, usually in capsule form, to see if an allergic response occurs.

Warning: Some people put themselves on highly restricted diets without proper medical consultation. This can result in serious nutritional deficiencies; it is best to consult a doctor.

LIVING WITH ALLERGIES

Once the offending allergens have been identified, eliminating those foods from the diet should solve the problem. But this can be more complicated than it sounds. Some of the most common food allergens, such as milk, eggs, wheat, and corn, are hidden ingredients in many processed foods (see Common Food Allergens and Their Symptoms, p.15). When you shop, scrutinize all food labels carefully. Also, many foods are chemically related; thus, a person allergic to lemons may also be allergic to oranges and other citrus fruits. In some cases, the real culprit may be a contaminant or an accidental additive in food. For example, some people who are allergic to orange juice and other citrus juices may actually be able to tolerate the peeled fruits themselves, since it is limonene, the oil in citrus peels, that often produces the allergic reaction. Some people only experience food allergy symptoms if they consume the offending food just before exercising.

Eating out can pose a few problems. When invited to someone's home, let your host know in advance if you are allergic to specific foods. Or ask about the menu; if it presents problems, offer to bring a substitute dish for yourself. Usually, however, it's sufficient to make inquiries upon arrival and then quietly decline the problem dishes.

In restaurants, ask servers about food ingredients before ordering. If they are unable to answer your questions, ask that they be directed to the chef. In order to avoid potential allergens, some people will have to select simple, ungarnished dishes, such as unseasoned broiled fish, a baked potato, and steamed vegetables. Or call the restaurant ahead of time to request that food be specially prepared.

TREATING EMERGENCIES

If you have had—or your doctor believes you are susceptible to—severe hives, asthma attacks, or anaphylactic reactions, you should always wear a medical identification pendant or carry

RISK-FREE FOODS. *Experts believe that some foods, including those pictured below, seldom if ever set off allergic reactions.*

emergency medical information in your wallet or purse. Your doctor may also recommend that you carry antihistamine medication or an easy-to-inject form of epinephrine (Adrenalin) to use in case of breathing problems or another severe allergic reaction.

A DIFFERENT PROBLEM

Many people mistakenly assume they have food allergies when, in fact, the problem is intolerance. The symptoms may be similar, but an allergic reaction is mediated through the immune system, whereas food intolerance originates in the gastrointestinal system and entails an inability to digest or absorb certain substances.

One of the most common types is lactose intolerance, in which a person lacks an enzyme (lactase) needed to digest milk sugar. The degree of lactose intolerance varies in different people. In severe cases even a tiny amount of milk sugar may provoke symptoms—generally abdominal pain and bloating, diarrhea, and flatulence. However, lactose-reduced dairy products are available, as are tablets that can be taken before eating; these have the enzyme that makes digesting dairy products possible. In contrast, a person who is allergic to milk will still have symptoms after ingesting even lactose-free milk products.

ALZHEIMER'S DISEASE

EAT PLENTY OF

- *Eggs, liver, soybeans and soy products, whole grains, brewer's yeast, and wheat germ—all reasonably good sources of lecithin and choline.*

AVOID

- *Zinc supplements, which may hasten the onset of symptoms.*
- *Alcohol, which can worsen memory loss and dementia.*

Alzheimer's disease is the leading cause of dementia in people over the age of 65, affecting some 300,000 Canadians. There are no specific diagnostic tests for Alzheimer's, but before arriving at a diagnosis, tests are needed to rule out a stroke, a brain tumor, nutritional deficiencies, thyroid disorders, syphilis, and other possible causes of dementia.

The cause of Alzheimer's disease remains unknown, but researchers theorize that chromosomal and genetic factors are responsible for many cases. The increased incidence of Alzheimer's among people with Down's syndrome, which is caused by a chromosomal abnormality, seems to support this theory. Researchers have discovered a genetic marker, a type of lipoprotein that can be detected by blood tests, that identifies people likely to develop the disease.

In addition, hormonal factors are under study. Women are afflicted more often than men; some recent studies indicate that estrogen replacement may protect against Alzheimer's. Thyroid disorders are also linked to an increased risk of the disease. The long-term use of nonsteroidal anti-inflammatory drugs (NSAIDs) has been linked with a reduced incidence of the disease.

There have been other intriguing leads, but researchers have been unable to pinpoint any specific dietary factors that increase the risk of or help to prevent Alzheimer's disease. Over the years, some research has implicated aluminum, which has been found in the abnormal tangles of brain cells in some Alzheimer's patients. However, extensive studies have failed to prove that aluminum actually causes the disease, and most experts now discount it as a factor. Still, some people believe it is prudent to avoid taking antacids with large amounts of aluminum or using cookware that allows the metal to leach into food. Concern has also been raised about the aluminum content of drinking water in areas where aluminum compounds are used as flocculating agents in municipal water treatment.

DIET AND ALZHEIMER'S

Researchers now think that a buildup of zinc may be a more relevant factor than aluminum; laboratory experiments show that zinc can transform the protein in brain cells into abnormal tangles indistinguishable from those of Alzheimer's. Other studies indicate that taking high-dose zinc supplements may hasten the progression of memory loss and other manifestations of the disease.

People with Alzheimer's disease have abnormally low levels of choline acetyltransferase, an enzyme necessary to make acetylcholine, a brain chemical believed to be instrumental in learning and memory. Also, the brain cells most affected by Alzheimer's are those that normally respond to acetylcholine. In addition, tacrine (Cognex), a new drug that appears to improve the memory of some Alzheimer's patients, increases levels of acetylcholine. Some nutrition researchers theorize that supplements or foods high in lecithin or choline (the major component of acetylcholine) can also slow the progression of Alzheimer's by raising acetylcholine production. So far, studies have failed to document its value, but some nutritionists feel that foods high in lecithin and choline may

help forestall Alzheimer's symptoms and will certainly do no harm; these include egg yolks, organ meats, soy products, wheat germ, and whole grains.

As Alzheimer's disease progresses, its victims may forget to eat or may limit their diets to sweets or other favorite foods. These patients should be persuaded to eat nutritionally balanced meals. They may even need to be spoon-fed if they have difficulty feeding themselves. A multivitamin supplement may also be advisable; however, high-dose supplements should not be administered unless specifically recommended by a physician. Contrary to media reports, there is no proof that high doses of vitamin E benefit Alzheimer's patients.

Even in small amounts, alcohol destroys brain cells, a loss that a healthy person can tolerate but one that can accelerate the progression of Alzheimer's disease. Alcohol interacts with antidepressants, sedatives, and other medications prescribed for Alzheimer's patients. It's a good idea to withhold all alcohol from persons with the disease.

ANEMIA

EAT PLENTY OF

- *Organ meats, beef and other meats, poultry, fish, and egg yolks for iron and vitamin B₁₂.*
- *Dried beans and peas, tofu and other soy products, dates, raisins, dried apricots, and blackstrap molasses—all good plant sources of iron.*
- *Iron-enriched breads and cereals.*
- *Citrus fruits and other good sources of vitamin C, which increase the body's iron absorption.*
- *Green leafy vegetables for folate.*

CUT DOWN ON

- *Bran, spinach, and rhubarb, which hinder iron absorption.*
- *Zinc and calcium supplements, antacids, coffee, and tea, which also reduce iron absorption.*

AVOID

- *Iron supplements, unless prescribed by a physician.*

Anemia is the umbrella term for a variety of disorders that are characterized by the inability of red blood cells to carry sufficient oxygen. This may be due to an abnormality in the shape or composition of the cells or a deficiency in their number. One of the common abnormalities is a low level of hemoglobin, the iron- and protein-based red pigment in blood that carries oxygen from the lungs to all body cells. Symptoms of anemia, therefore, reflect oxygen starvation. In mild anemia, this may include general weakness, pallor, fatigue, and brittle, spoon-shaped nails. More severe cases are marked by shortness of breath, fainting, and cardiac arrhythmias.

IRON-DEFICIENCY ANEMIA

In Canada the most common type of anemia is due to iron deficiency, which is usually caused by massive or chronic

Case Study

After weeks of feeling tired and short of breath, Roy, a retired librarian, went for a checkup. Blood studies showed that Roy was anemic, and a stool test indicated hidden intestinal bleeding was the likely cause. Roy's doctor sent him for a colonoscopy, which revealed a suspicious growth in the uppermost segment of the bowel. A biopsy confirmed that the growth was cancerous.

In preparation for colon surgery 3 weeks later, the doctor prescribed iron pills to help build up Roy's hemoglobin levels. The surgeon removed the diseased segment of Roy's colon and rejoined the healthy portions. The cancer was in an early stage, so bowel function returned to normal within 10 days. Because he was still anemic, Roy was instructed to take iron pills for another 3 months and to eat a diet of iron-rich foods.

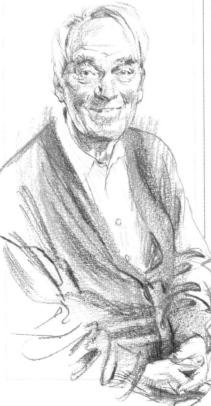

blood loss. Surgery patients, accident victims, or people with a bleeding ulcer or intestinal cancer often have iron-deficiency anemia. In fact, a blood test that shows iron deficiency often prompts a physician to investigate the possibility of colon cancer. Women with heavy menstrual periods, especially adolescents, are at risk.

Dietary iron deficiency is relatively uncommon in Canada because the typical diet—high in meat and iron-enriched breads and cereal—usually provides more than enough iron for most people. Some exceptions, however, are infants and young children who drink mostly milk; pregnant women because they need extra iron for their developing fetus and their own expanded blood volume. Vegetarians, too, may become iron deficient; as may people with inflammatory disorders.

OTHER TYPES OF ANEMIA

Hemolytic anemia occurs when red blood cells are destroyed more rapidly than normal. The cause may be hereditary or one of a variety of diseases, including leukemia and other cancers, abnormal spleen function, autoimmune disorders, and severe hypertension.

Pernicious, or megaloblastic, anemia is caused by a deficiency of vitamin B₁₂, which is necessary to make red blood cells. This deficiency can result from a vegetarian diet that eschews all animal products, but the most common cause is an intestinal disorder that prevents absorption of the vitamin.

Deficiency of folate, another B vitamin, can also cause anemia in pregnant women (who need extra folate for the developing fetus), in alcoholics, and in elderly people.

Relatively rare types of anemia include thalassemia, an inherited disorder, and aplastic anemia, which may be caused by infection, exposure to toxic chemicals or radiation, or a genetic disorder.

HOW MUCH IRON DO YOU NEED?

The human body recycles iron to make new red blood cells. Even so, the body loses an average of 1mg for men and 1.5mg for women during their reproductive years. The body absorbs only a small percentage of dietary iron, so the Recommended Nutrient Intakes (RNIs) call for consuming more than what is lost: 9mg a day for adult men and post-menopausal women, 13mg for women under 50 and for pregnant women, with an additional 5mg during the second trimester, and an additional 10mg during the third trimester.

Those who have nutrition-related anemias can benefit from a session with a registered dietitian or a qualified nutritionist to help structure a more healthful diet. The best sources of iron are animal products—meat, fish, poultry, and egg yolks. The body absorbs much more of the heme iron found in these foods than the nonheme iron from plant sources, such as green leafy vegetables, dried fruits, soy and other legumes, and iron-enriched breads and cereals. Combining iron-rich foods with citrus or other fruits and vegetables high in vitamin C increases iron absorption; conversely, antacids and bran bind with iron and prevent the body from using it.

Cooking tomatoes and other acidic foods in iron pots can add large amounts of iron to food. For example, 4 ounces of tomato sauce provides 0.7mg of iron; cooking it in an iron pot adds 5mg. Foods cooked in ironware may be discolored, but the taste is unaffected.

ANOREXIA NERVOSA

TAKE

- *At least a small amount of a variety of nutritious foods.*
- *Multivitamin pills and calorie-enriched liquid supplements if approved by a doctor.*

AVOID

- *Coffee, diet soft drinks, and low-calorie diet foods.*
- *Appetite suppressants, diuretics, and laxatives.*

The self-starvation that is a hallmark of anorexia nervosa is caused by a complex psychiatric disorder that afflicts between 1 and 2 percent of Canadians, mostly adolescent girls or, less commonly, young women. (Only about 5 percent of anorexics are males; they are often weight-conscious adolescent boys who are dancers or athletes.)

The cause of anorexia—a medical term for appetite loss—is unknown. Researchers believe that a combination of hormonal, social, and psychological factors are responsible. The disease often begins in adolescence, a time of tremendous hormonal and psychological change. Convinced that she is too fat, regardless of how much she weighs, the girl begins obsessive dieting. Some girls adopt a very restricted diet. Others become overly preoccupied with food, often planning and preparing elaborate meals that they then refuse to eat. And when the anorexic does eat, she may resort to self-induced vomiting or laxative abuse to avoid gaining weight. Many anorexics also exercise obsessively, often for several hours a day.

As the disease progresses, menstruation ceases and nutritional deficiencies develop. Many anorexics try to hide their thinness by wearing oversized clothes; physical indications of anorexia include fatigue, nervousness or hyperactivity, dry skin, hair loss, and intolerance to cold. More serious consequences include cardiac arrhythmias, loss of bone mass, kidney failure, and in about 15 percent of cases, death.

TREATMENT STRATEGIES

Anorexia often requires intensive long-term treatment, preferably by a team experienced with eating disorders: a doctor to treat starvation-induced medical problems, a psychiatrist, and a dietitian. Family members can also benefit from counseling.

Anorexics tend to be defensive about their eating habits and resistant to treatment. Most anorexics are treated on an outpatient basis, but in severe cases, hospitalization and intravenous nutritional therapy are necessary.

The biggest hurdle is to help the anorexic overcome her abnormal fear of food and distorted self-image of being fat. Counseling is directed to uncovering the source of these fears.

In the beginning, the patient is offered small portions of nutritious and easily digestible foods, perhaps eggs, custards, soups, and milk shakes. Portion sizes and the variety of foods are increased gradually to achieve a steady weight gain. This does not require huge amounts of food; instead, doctors strive for a varied diet that provides adequate protein for rebuilding lost lean tissue, carbohydrate for energy, and a moderate amount of fat for extra calories. Extra calcium and a multivitamin pill may also be given.

Because an anorexic is skilled at deceiving others about her eating and relapses are common, close monitoring may be necessary to make sure that she is really eating. But avoid making food a constant source of attention and conflict; group therapy can be more helpful than parental nagging.

ANTIOXIDANTS: SORTING THROUGH FACTS AND HYPE

Since oxygen is essential for life, it's ironic that its use by the body sets the stage for aging and many diseases. The good news is that antioxidants in foods seem to stave off these effects.

Similar to the oxygen requirements of a burning fire, every cell in your body needs a steady supply of oxygen to derive energy from digested food. But consuming oxygen comes with a price; it also releases free radicals, unstable molecules that can damage healthy cells as they career through the body. Free radicals are highly reactive because they contain an unpaired electron in search of a mate. As soon as these radicals are formed, they search for molecules with which they can react, or oxidize. Oxidation in this sense refers to a process by which a molecule loses electrons.

Although all healthy cells produce small amounts of free radicals, excessive bombardment by these molecules damages cellular DNA and other genetic material. However, human cells have protective enzymes that repair 99 percent of oxidative damage. But oxygen metabolism is not the only source of oxidative damage; it can come from X-rays, ultraviolet rays, radon, tobacco smoke, and other environmental pollutants. The cumulative effect can cause irreversible cellular changes, or mutations, that can result in cancer and other diseases.

The body's immune system seeks out and destroys these mutated cells, in much the same way as it eliminates

---

BENEFITS

- *Protect against cancer, heart disease, cataracts, and other degenerative diseases.*
- *May slow the aging process.*
- *Prevent the spoilage of oils and processed foods.*

DRAWBACKS

- *May have detrimental effects if taken as high-dose supplements.*

---

invading bacteria and other foreign organisms; this mechanism lessens with age, however. The body becomes more vulnerable to free-radical damage, and the incidence of degenerative disorders increases. Consequences range from harmless pigmented skin patches to more serious disorders, such as cataracts, cancer, and a host of degenerative diseases.

Antioxidants are molecules that combine with free radicals, rendering them harmless. The major antioxidants are vitamins C and E; beta carotene, which the body converts to vitamin A; and selenium. Bioflavonoids, substances found in citrus fruits, grapes, and other fresh fruits and vegetables, have antioxidant properties, as do some other phyto-

---

ANTIOXIDANT PANTRY. *Fresh fruits and vegetables, fatty fish, nuts, legumes, and various vegetable oils are rich sources of antioxidants.*

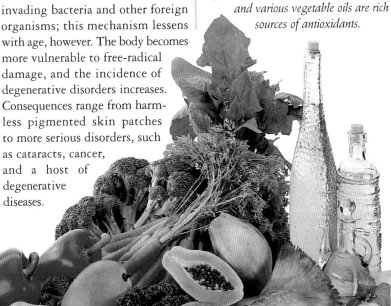

20

chemicals, that is, substances which are found in plants.

Numerous studies show a reduced incidence of cancer and heart attacks in people who eat plenty of fruits, vegetables, and whole-grain products— the best food sources of antioxidants. Recent research indicates that antioxidants such as vitamin E may prevent heart disease by hindering the oxidation of LDLs (low-density lipoproteins), the harmful cholesterol. Unoxidized LDLs are relatively benign, but after oxidation they promote atherosclerosis, the development of artery-clogging plaque. Oxidation also facilitates the uptake of LDLs into artery walls; a process that may be blocked by beta carotene.

Less is known about how antioxidants hinder cancer; researchers theorize that prevention of DNA damage is a factor. Recent studies indicate that vitamin C may protect against skin cancer and melanoma.

ANTIOXIDANT PILLS

Doctors discourage taking high-dose antioxidant supplements. When taken in large amounts, some nutrients that are normally antioxidants may have the opposite effect and actually increase oxidation. For example, when taken by someone who has large iron reserves, high doses of vitamin C become pro-oxidant. Similarly, recent studies failed to find any benefit from high-dose beta carotene supplements and even suggested that they could lead to an increased risk of lung cancer in smokers.

Supplements exceeding the RNIs should be taken only under medical supervision. High doses of vitamin E, for example, can interfere with blood clotting and increase the risk of a bleeding emergency. Even so, supplements may be prescribed for some heart patients, because it is impossible to get protective amounts (200mg to 400mg a day) from diet alone.

PROTECTIVE PLANT CHEMICALS

Because plants are also susceptible to disease, they have developed their own protective substances, called phytochemicals (from phyton, *the Greek term for* plant*). Mounting research shows that many phytochemicals also protect humans against cancer and other diseases.*

PHYTO-CHEMICAL	FUNCTIONS	SOURCES
Allylic sulfides	May stimulate production of protective enzymes.	Garlic, onions
Bioflavonoids	Antioxidant; inhibit cancer-promoting hormones.	Most fresh fruits and vegetables
Catechins (tannins)	Antioxidant.	Berries, green tea
Curcumin	Protects against tobacco-induced carcinogens.	Turmeric, cumin
Genistein	Inhibits tumor growth.	Soybeans
Indoles	Inhibit estrogen, which stimulates some cancers; induce protective enzymes.	Broccoli, cabbage, cauliflower, mustard greens
Isoflavones	Block estrogen uptake by cancer cells.	Beans, peanuts and other legumes, peas
Isothiocyanates	Induce production of protective enzymes.	Horseradish, mustard, radishes
Lignans	Inhibit estrogen and block prostaglandins.	Flaxseed, walnuts
Lycopene	Antioxidant; may protect against prostate cancer.	Pink grapefruit, tomatoes, watermelon
Monoterpenes	Some antioxidant properties; aid in activity of protective enzymes.	Basil, citrus fruits, broccoli, orange and yellow vegetables
Omega-3 fatty acids	Inhibit estrogen; reduce inflammation.	Canola oil, flaxseed, walnuts, fatty fish
Phenolic acids	Inhibit nitrosamines; enhance enzyme activity.	Berries, broccoli, cabbage, carrots, citrus fruits, eggplant, parsley, peppers, teas, tomatoes, whole grains
Protease inhibitors	Suppress production of enzymes in cancer cells.	Soybeans
Quercetin	Inhibits cellular mutation, carcinogens, clot formation, and inflammation.	Grape skins, red and white wine, tea
Sulforaphane	Induces protective enzymes.	Broccoli
Terpenes	Stimulate anticancer enzymes.	Citrus fruits

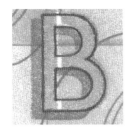

BAD BREATH

CONSUME PLENTY OF
- *Water, fruit juice, and sour foods to stimulate saliva flow.*

CUT DOWN ON
- *Sticky sweet foods to reduce plaque.*

AVOID
- *Garlic, onions, and other foods that have strong odors.*
- *Alcohol and tobacco products, which give the breath an unpleasant odor.*
- *Drugs that cause dry mouth.*

Halitosis, the transient bad breath that everyone develops occasionally, is usually a trivial problem caused by certain foods or drinks, smoking, or poor dental hygiene. Often, a chemical in food is responsible. The bad breath caused by eating onions and garlic, for example, is due to a number of smelly sulfur compounds they contain. Residues of wine, beer, and other alcoholic drinks produce a breath odor; and tobacco in any form makes the breath smell stale.

Saliva controls the mouth's bacteria population. A drop in saliva production, such as during sleep or the natural decline with age, allows bacteria, especially at the back of the tongue, to multiply and form plaque. This scenario accounts for morning breath and the bad breath experienced by many older people. More persistent dry mouth may require treatment with artificial saliva, sold at drugstores.

Most bad breath can be remedied by good dental hygiene, eliminating the offending foods from the diet, and abstaining from alcohol and tobacco. If bad breath persists despite these measures, see your dentist first and, if no cause is found, your physician next.

Persistent bad breath may be a sign of an underlying illness. Some diseases, such as kidney failure, liver disease, and diabetes, cause certain odors. Other problems that can cause bad breath include tonsillitis, sinus and nasal problems, bronchitis and other respiratory infections, and some cancers. Disorders that reduce the flow of saliva, such as lupus, also cause bad breath.

QUICK FIXES

Mild bad breath can be camouflaged with a commercial mouth rinse or with foods or herbs that mask the odor. For example, chewing a few sprigs of parsley or peppermint, or anise, dill, or fennel seeds quickly freshens breath. Some people report good results from commercially available pills made from parsley seeds (Breath-asure).

Antiseptic mouth rinses control bad breath by reducing oral bacteria; products with chlorine dioxide are effective. Nonantiseptic rinses simply mask the odor. To make your own rinse, steep three whole (or ¼ teaspoon ground) cloves in hot water for 20 minutes. A commercial toothpaste with fluoride, baking soda, and hydrogen peroxide cleans the teeth and freshens the breath. To make your own, add a few drops of hydrogen peroxide to baking soda.

BANANAS

BENEFITS
- *A good source of potassium, folate, and vitamins C and B₆.*

Healthful, filling, and tasty, bananas are one of nature's ideal snacks. The fruit, which is grown in most of the world's tropical areas, is harvested while still green. When stored at room temperature, most bananas ripen in a few days; the process can be hastened, however, by placing them in a plastic or paper bag along with an apple.

Because bananas are bland, easy to digest, and hypoallergenic, they are an ideal early food for babies. Bananas, along with rice, applesauce, and toast, are one of the foods in the BRAT diet recommended after a bout of diarrhea. Some ulcer patients report that bananas alleviate some of their pain, but this is unproven.

NUTRITIONAL VALUE

Bananas are exceeded only by avocados (which are high in fat) as a fruit source for potassium, a mineral instrumental in proper muscle function. Patients taking certain diuretic drugs for high blood pressure are usually advised to eat two or three bananas a day to help replace the potassium lost in the urine.

A relatively good source of vitamin B_6, a medium (4-ounce) banana supplies one-third the Recommended Nutrient Intake (RNI), along with 10 percent or more of the RNIs for vitamin C and folate. It adds 2g of soluble dietary fiber, which helps to lower blood cholesterol levels. Bananas contain about 100 calories each, mostly in the form of fruit sugar and starch. Because the body quickly converts these to energy, they are a favorite of athletes.

PLANTAINS

These resemble large green bananas, but they never become as sweet. Plantains are baked or fried and served as a starchy side dish; they can also be a delicious addition to soups, stews, and meat dishes. Nutritionally, plantains are comparable to bananas, except that their content of vitamin A is much higher, providing approximately 20 percent of the RNI.

BASIC FOOD GROUPS

The athlete who burns thousands of calories a day and the somewhat sedentary retiree are poles apart in their energy needs. Still, both require the same balance of nutrients to stay healthy.

The essence of a healthy diet can be summed up with three words: variety, moderation, and balance. To make it easy to follow these simple principles, Health Canada has devised the Food Guide Rainbow (see below), which divides foods into four basic groups and recommends a number of daily servings for each. These servings are of moderate size, and if a person selects a variety of foods from each group, there should be no problem in achieving a balanced diet. Still, even those who try to follow the Food Guide guidelines frequently find that they have ques-

5 GUIDELINES FOR HEALTHY EATING

In addition to the Food Guide Rainbow, Health Canada has established the following guidelines for healthy Canadians:

1. Enjoy a variety of foods.

2. Emphasize cereals, breads, other grain products, vegetables, and fruits.

3. Choose lower-fat dairy products, leaner meats, and foods prepared with little or no fat.

4. Achieve and maintain a healthy body weight by enjoying regular physical activity and healthy eating.

5. Limit salt, alcohol, and caffeine.

tions: "Where do fast foods like pizza fit in?," "Won't 12 servings of starchy grains a day cause me to gain weight?," and "Do these guidelines lower my cholesterol?"

THE NEED FOR VARIETY

To maintain health, the body needs a proper balance of carbohydrates, fats, and proteins for energy, growth, and repair or replacement of damaged cells. Also essential to maintain health are at least 13 vitamins and 16 minerals. Nutrition researchers believe that there are still other essential nutrients that have not yet been identified. Although it is not a nutrient, water—the most abundant sub-

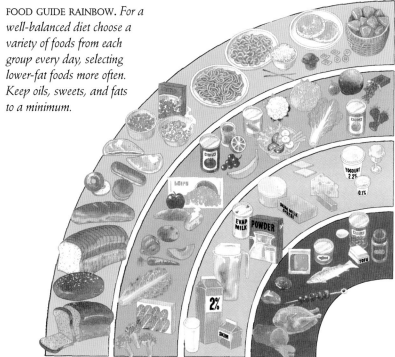

FOOD GUIDE RAINBOW. *For a well-balanced diet choose a variety of foods from each group every day, selecting lower-fat foods more often. Keep oils, sweets, and fats to a minimum.*

Grain Products. Have 5 to 12 servings per day. Choose whole grain and enriched products more often.

Vegetables and Fruit. Have 5 to 10 servings per day. Choose dark green and orange vegetables and orange fruit more often.

Milk Products. Have 2 to 4 servings per day. Choose lower-fat milk products more often.

Meat & Alternatives. Have 2 to 3 servings per day. Choose leaner meats, poultry and fish, as well as dried peas, beans and lentils more often.

THE FOOD GROUPS: TAKING THE PATH TO HEALTHIER EATING

A balanced diet emphasizes a wide variety of grains and other complex carbohydrates, vegetables, fruits, and smaller amounts of meat and fish, dairy products, and fats. The chart below lists *the recommended daily amounts, in descending order, for the four Food Guide Rainbow groups (see Food Guide Rainbow, p.23), and suggests ways to improve your diet.*

FOOD GROUPS AND THEIR NUTRIENTS	TRY TO	AVOID
GRAIN PRODUCTS 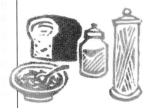 **5 to 12 servings daily.** These foods provide complex carbohydrates (starches) and are a major source of B vitamins, magnesium, and many other minerals; enriched breads and cereals also provide iron; some products have been fortified with calcium.	Whenever possible, use whole-grain products. Combine grains with beans and other legumes to make a low-fat complete protein.	Frying any of the foods in this group. In addition, use butter, margarine, and other types of creamy spreads and sauces only in moderation.
VEGETABLES **3 to 5 servings daily.** An assortment of these foods provides fiber and numerous vitamins and minerals, including vitamins A and C, folate, potassium, and magnesium, and they supply important plant chemicals that prevent tumor growth. 	Include servings of broccoli, Brussels sprouts, cabbage, and other cruciferous vegetables 3 or 4 times a week. These foods, along with yellow or orange vegetables, contain protective bioflavonoids.	Frying vegetables in oil and with batter; serving with butter or cream sauces; overcooking, which destroys some nutrients.
FRUITS **2 to 5 servings daily.** Like vegetables, fruits offer a broad range of nutrients, including beta carotene, vitamin C, potassium, fiber, and various bioflavonoids and other beneficial plant chemicals. 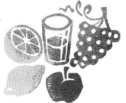	Eat a broad spectrum of fruits, including at least one citrus fruit per day. Incorporate them into your meals and eat them as snacks instead of products that are high in fat and sugar.	Consuming all fruit servings at once. Too much acidic food may lead to intestinal upsets.
MILK PRODUCTS 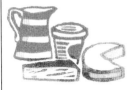 **2 to 4 servings daily.** Dairy products—such as milk, cheeses, yogurt, and other milk products—are the main source of calcium. They also provide protein and riboflavin and other B vitamins.	Opt for low-fat versions of dairy products, such as milk (skim or 1% fat), yogurt, and cheese. Look for brands that have been fortified with vitamins A and D.	Products or recipes that contain heavy cream, butter, whole milk, or full-fat cheese.
MEAT AND ALTERNATIVES **2 to 3 servings daily.** This group provides the bulk of dietary protein, as well as the B vitamins, iron, phosphorus, magnesium, zinc, and other minerals. 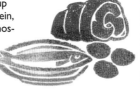	Opt for poultry or fish. Limit red meats and fatty or processed meats, such as sausage and bologna; instead, choose lean meats and trim all fat before cooking.	Frying or sautéeing in fat; instead, cook by grilling, baking, roasting, or stir-frying.
OTHER FOODS 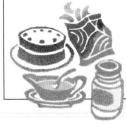 **Use sparingly.** This group includes margarine, butter, oils, sugar, chocolate, and other sweet or fatty foods. Only a very small amount of fat is necessary for the body to function properly.	Emphasize monounsaturated fats, such as canola and olive oils. Flavor with spices instead of frying in oils or using fatty spreads. Skim fat from meat juices, stews, and soups.	Fatty snack foods, such as potato chips, chocolate, pastries, and ice cream.

stance in the human body—is also essential to sustain life.

Keeping track of the daily intake of the more than 30 known essential nutrients is a daunting, if not impossible, task; fortunately, there's no need to do so. By consuming sensible portions from each of the food groups, most people will get all the nutrients that they need.

THE BASIC FOOD GROUPS

In Canada, public nutrition education is looked after by Health and Welfare Canada. Canada's Food Guide divides common foods into four categories: grain products, milk products, fruits and vegetables, and meat and alternatives.

The Food Guide describes the number and size of servings that should be consumed from each food group, making allowances for pregnant and breast-feeding women, males and females, age, body size, and activity level. Following the general concepts will result in a "nutritious diet." This means that energy needs will be fulfilled, micronutrient requirements (vitamins and minerals) will be met, and the macronutrients (proteins, fats, and carbohydrates) will be consumed in an appropriate ratio.

The optimal balance is arrived at by featuring an abundance of servings from the grain and fruit and vegetable groups, while limiting intake of fattier foods found in the milk and meat categories. If the guidelines are followed, no more than 30 percent of the total number of calories will come from fats.

The total number of servings a day adds up to a minimum of 14 and a maximum of 29, which sounds like a lot, but portions are quite small (see What Makes a Serving?, above) and the number of servings should be adjusted according to individual energy needs. A truly balanced diet is one that provides all the essential nutrients

WHAT MAKES A SERVING?

FOOD GROUP	SAMPLE SERVING
Grain products	1 slice bread; $\frac{1}{2}$ bagel, pita or bun; $\frac{1}{2}$ cup pasta or rice; 1 bowl of hot cereal; 1 bowl of cold cereal
Vegetables	$\frac{1}{2}$ cup fresh, frozen, or canned vegetables; 1 medium-size vegetable; 1 cup salad; $\frac{1}{2}$ cup juice
Fruits	$\frac{1}{2}$ cup fresh, frozen, or canned fruit; 1 medium-size fruit; $\frac{1}{2}$ cup juice
Milk products	1 cup milk; $\frac{3}{4}$ cup yogurt; $1\frac{1}{2}$ oz of cheese
Meat and alternatives	2 to 3 oz lean meat, poultry, or fish; $\frac{1}{3}$ to $\frac{2}{3}$ can of fish; 1 to 2 eggs; $\frac{1}{3}$ cup of tofu; 2 tbsp of peanut butter

while maintaining the ideal body weight. Thus, a person trying to shed a few pounds may have the maximum number of low-calorie fruits and vegetables and the minimum number of servings from the meat, dairy, and starch groups, which tend to be higher in calories.

RECOMMENDED NUTRIENT INTAKES (RNIs)

To meet the nutritional needs of most people, the Nutrition Research Division of Health and Welfare Canada established the Recommended Nutrient Intakes, or RNIs, for 9 vitamins, 6 minerals, protein, and energy.

The Nutrition Research Division also lists the estimated safe and adequate intakes of two other vitamins and five minerals. To determine a specific RNI, nutrition scientists establish a minimum value, below which deficiency develops, and a maximum amount, above which harm might occur. The RNI is set between these two values, with a margin of safety to ensure a reserve to carry a person through weeks or even months of inadequate intake.

Many people mistakenly assume that they must consume the full RNI of each nutrient daily. This is not true, because each RNI is actually more than a person needs. For example,

the RNI for vitamin C (40mg) is really four times what the average person needs to prevent scurvy. It should be noted that in Canada, deficiency diseases are rare, occurring mostly among people with other disorders—for example, thiamine deficiency is common among long-term alcoholics and the elderly.

THE MEDITERRANEAN DIET

Observing that the people of Greece, Italy, and other Mediterranean countries have much lower cholesterol levels and far fewer heart attacks than North Americans, researchers have tried to determine why. Many have concluded that the answer lies in their diet.

In contrast to the typical North American diet, wine is a regular feature of the Mediterranean diet. The bulk of the diet consists of pasta, bread, grains and other starches, fresh fruits and vegetables, nuts and beans.

Consumed regularly, about every other day, are cheese and yogurt, olives and olive oil. Sweets, eggs, poultry and fish are served frequently, a few times a week. Least often consumed is red meat, which is typically served in small portions, only a few times each month.

Although the Mediterranean diet does not specify serving sizes, as a general rule of thumb Western nutritionists recommend eating more pasta, grains, breads, fruits and vegetables, legumes, yogurt, cheese, and olives or olive oil, and less poultry and fish, sweets, eggs, and especially red meat.

More than 30 percent of total calories in the typical Mediterranean diet come from fats, mostly monounsaturated olive oil. Nutritionists note that the diet provides more fat and calories than what is generally recommended for most North Americans, but because so many Mediterranean people have physically demanding occupations, they are less likely to gain weight.

THE QUESTION OF SUPPLEMENTS

Millions of people take high-dose vitamin pills daily, especially beta carotene and vitamins C and E, the ANTIOXIDANT nutrients that have received so much media attention in recent years. But supplements are no substitute for good eating habits, and the vast majority of people can fulfill their nutritional needs by following the Food Guide Rainbow (see p.23).

Megadose supplements can actually be harmful. When taken in very large amounts, vitamins and minerals, like all drugs, carry a risk of adverse side effects and interactions. Many minerals, and vitamins A and D, are stored in the body and can build to toxic levels when taken in excess. The presence of large quantities of a particular vitamin or mineral in the intestinal tract invariably interferes with the body's absorption of other nutrients and can actually lead to deficiency diseases.

If supplements are needed, they should only be prescribed by a doctor. For example, a woman planning to conceive or who is already pregnant needs extra folate to protect her baby from neurological problems. Pregnancy also increases the demand for iron beyond what can be obtained from an ordinary diet. An older woman may need additional calcium and vitamin D to help prevent osteoporosis.

HOW MUCH WATER DO WE NEED?

A healthy adult needs 2½ to 3 quarts of fluids a day. Some of this fluid comes from food, but six to eight glasses should come from water or other nonalcoholic drinks (avoid drinks high in sugar and caffeine). Prolonged exercise, hot weather, diarrhea, and a fever are among many conditions that demand extra fluid intake. In these cases drink extra fluids before signs of thirst occur (thirst is unreliable, especially in the elderly).

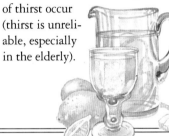

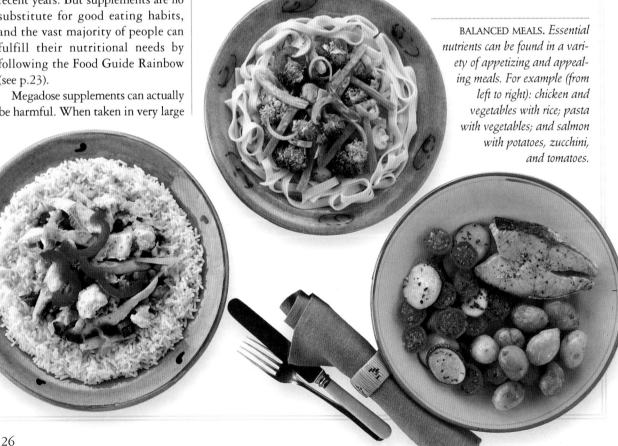

BALANCED MEALS. *Essential nutrients can be found in a variety of appetizing and appealing meals. For example (from left to right): chicken and vegetables with rice; pasta with vegetables; and salmon with potatoes, zucchini, and tomatoes.*

BEANS

BENEFITS

- *High in folate and vitamins A and C.*
- *Mature (shelled) beans are high in protein and iron.*

DRAWBACKS

- *Shelled beans can cause flatulence.*
- *Fava beans are toxic to some people.*

Green beans (which can also be yellow or purple) are harvested at an immature stage. Both the tender pods and small, soft seeds are eaten. In shelled varieties only the seeds are eaten. Some, such as lima beans, are harvested while they are still tender; others are left to mature. Most pod beans—snap beans, Italian green beans, long Chinese beans, purple and yellow wax beans, and green beans—can be eaten raw. More commonly, they are steamed or boiled. Shelled beans should always be cooked; they can be served hot or cold.

NUTRITIONAL VALUE

Limas and favas are good sources of protein, providing about 7g per half-cup serving. The same-size serving of baby or green lima beans contains 2mg of iron, more than twice as much as in favas and four times the amount in ½ cup of green snap beans. All these varieties are good sources of folate and vitamins A and C. Shelled beans have more thiamine, vitamin B_6, potassium, and magnesium; the soluble fiber in shelled beans may lower cholesterol, but the presence of carbohydrates such as raffinose may also cause flatulence.

Warning: Some Mediterranean people lack an enzyme needed to protect red blood cells from damage by vicine, a toxic substance in fava beans that causes a type of anemia. People taking monoamine oxidase (MAO) inhibitors to treat depression should also avoid fava beans; the combination can raise blood pressure.

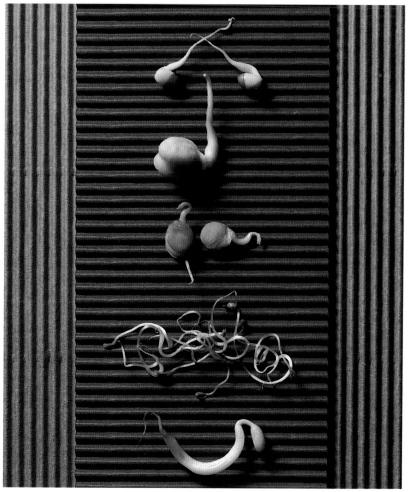

SPROUTING BEANS. *Among the most popular sprouts that can be grown at home are (from top to bottom) mung beans, chickpeas, green lentils, alfalfa, and soybeans.*

BEAN SPROUTS

BENEFITS

- *Some are high in folate; others are fair to good sources of protein, vitamin C, B vitamins, and iron.*

DRAWBACK

- *Alfalfa sprouts may provoke a flare-up of symptoms in lupus patients.*

Various types of sprouts are available in health-food stores, supermarkets, and salad bars. However, few live up to their reputation as the prototype of health foods. Some sprouts are much more nutritious than others. A cup of raw mung bean sprouts, for example, provides one-third of the Recommended Nutrient Intake (RNI) of folate and 30 percent of the RNI for vitamin C. In contrast, it takes approximately five cups of alfalfa sprouts to yield comparable amounts.

Warning: Most sprouts can be eaten raw. An important exception is the sprouted soybean, which contains a potentially harmful toxin that is destroyed by cooking. People with lupus should avoid alfalfa sprouts; alfalfa in any form can prompt a flare-up of symptoms.

BEEF AND VEAL

BENEFITS
- *Major sources of high-quality protein.*
- *Contain a wide range of nutrients, especially vitamin B_{12}, iron, and zinc.*

DRAWBACKS
- *Beef fat is highly saturated and can increase blood cholesterol levels and the risk of cardiovascular disease.*
- *A high-meat diet may raise the risk of colon cancer and other cancers.*
- *Rare beef is a source of E. coli and toxoplasmosis infections.*

Although its consumption has decreased dramatically in recent decades, beef is still a popular red meat. One of the most versatile meats, beef may be prepared by roasting, stewing, broiling, frying, and grilling. Beef, especially in the form of hamburgers, is the most common meat served in restaurants.

There is no question that beef is a highly nutritious food source; not only is it a leading source of high-quality protein, but a 4-ounce serving provides more than 100 percent of the Recommended Nutrient Intake (RNI) of vitamin B_{12}, an essential nutrient found only in animal products. Beef is also an excellent source of vitamin B_6, niacin, and riboflavin, as well as such essential minerals as iron and zinc.

A CASE OF LESS IS BEST

Beef's major nutritional drawback is the large amount of mostly saturated fat in many cuts, especially prime roasts and steaks. It is also a leading source of dietary cholesterol. Studies link a diet with large amounts of meat to an increased risk of heart attacks and certain cancers. Even well-trimmed lean beef has some hidden fat. Nonetheless, nutritionists stress that beef can be part of a healthful, low-fat diet if it is limited to small, fat-trimmed portions of round steak, brisket, and other lean cuts.

The way beef is cooked substantially affects its fat content. Trimming away all visible fat is an obvious beginning; roasting or broiling beef on a rack or spit allows the fat to drip free of the meat. Another approach is to cook stews and soups in advance, chill them so that the congealed fat can be removed easily, and then reheat before serving. Of course, controlling the size of the portion is important. A 16-ounce T-bone steak, rack of short ribs, or huge slab of prime rib roast each have 800 to 1,000 calories, with half or more of them coming from fat. In contrast, a modest 4-ounce serving of choice-cut eye of round provides about 200 calories, 70 of which come from fat.

The liver, kidneys, and other organ meats are the most concentrated source of iron and vitamins A and B_{12} in beef. At one time, women were urged to eat an occasional serving of liver to prevent iron-deficiency anemia. But enthusiasm for liver and other organ meats has been

---

ABOUT VEAL

Very young calves produce the delicate pink, low-fat meat of veal, which has always been considered a luxury meat in Canada. To ensure that the meat is fine grained and light textured, veal growers often resort to keeping calves confined in small, enclosed stalls or boxes, preventing them from eating grass. The calves are fed only milk, and after just a few weeks, the confined animals become painfully anemic. Media campaigns to raise public awareness of the cruel plight of veal calves has resulted in a sharp decline in veal consumption, which is now about 3 pounds per person a year compared to over 5 pounds a few decades ago.

---

dampened in recent years for several reasons: They are very high in fat and cholesterol, and they may further increase the risk of heart disease.

Another issue revolves around the fact that factory-reared animals are fed large amounts of antibiotics and hormones, which concentrate in the animals' liver. Some experts contend that these drug and hormone residues pose a health risk to humans who ingest them; others, however, insist that they are safe. Still, some countries cite these potential risks as a reason to bar the importation of Canadian and American beef.

A woman who consumes liver products frequently may store large amounts of vitamin A in her body. Although it is unlikely that this would endanger her health, it might cause serious birth defects if she becomes pregnant. This risk is compounded if the woman is also taking vitamin A supplements.

ANOTHER HEALTH ISSUE

Recent outbreaks of a deadly type of *E. coli* infection have been traced to contaminated beef. There are many strains of *E. coli* bacteria, including harmless ones that normally inhabit the human intestinal tract. But in 1982 researchers identified a different strain, later called 0157:H7, in the intestinal tract of cattle. This type of *E. coli* can easily invade meat during slaughtering. Grinding the contaminated beef further spreads the bacteria through the meat. The organism can survive in hamburgers and other contaminated beef that is served rare, so it's important to cook the meat thoroughly. When this strain of *E. coli* reaches the human intestinal tract, it can cause mild to severe diarrhea. More seriously, some people—especially children, the elderly, and individuals with weakened immune systems—develop hemolytic uremic syndrome, a life-threatening disorder characterized by the rapid destruction of red blood cells and kidney failure.

Recent studies indicate that approximately 55,000 North Americans are stricken with *E. coli* infections from beef each year. Although some infections have been traced to rare roast beef, and a few to unpasteurized milk, rare hamburgers are by far the most common source. Public health officials stress that virtually all beef-borne *E. coli* infections can be prevented by cooking beef, especially hamburger, until it is well-done, with no traces of pink, and by using only pasteurized milk.

SOCIAL ISSUES

The process of producing a pound of beef requires much more land and other resources than growing an equivalent amount of vegetable protein. Critics of our high beef consumption point to the increasing destruction of the Amazon rain forests, as well as our own ecological systems, to make room for more cattle ranching. The growing trend to raise meat animals in enclosed factories creates different environmental problems altogether—in particular, finding ways to dispose of animal waste without polluting our rivers and other natural resources.

BEER

BENEFITS
- *Is lower in alcohol concentrations than wine and hard liquor.*
- *Contains modest amounts of niacin, folate, vitamin B_6, and some minerals.*

DRAWBACKS
- *Overconsumption can cause unwanted weight gain and obesity.*
- *Heavy drinking can lead to inebriation and alcoholism.*
- *Causes feelings of aggression in some people.*

Historians believe that humans began to brew beer some time around 5000 B.C. in what is now Iraq and Egypt. Barley, the grain that still dominates beer brewing, was abundant in that region. Nonetheless, almost every society worldwide has independently developed ways of making beer from local cereal grains: African tribes use sprouted corn, millet, and sorghum; Russians turn rye bread into a low-alcohol beer called kvass; the Chinese and Japanese use rice; and South and Central American Indians rely on corn to make their respective beers.

THE BREWING PROCESS

Although many societies around the world continue to use their traditional methods to make beer, modern brewing is a scientific process that begins with malting to convert grain starch into sugar that will ferment. To do this, the grain is sprouted in order to activate enzymes that will eventually turn the starch into sugar. The precise methods vary according to the type of beer being produced, but at some point the germination is stopped, the sprouts are removed, and the malted grain is then prepared for mashing. The malt is heated slowly to allow the enzymes to continue converting starch into a sugary broth called wort. The grain is allowed to settle, and the wort is heated and filtered through it into the brewing kettles. (The grains are then rinsed and salvaged for livestock feed.)

Hops, which are dried flowers from the hop vine, are added to the wort, and the mixture is boiled and then strained. (The used hops are added to livestock feed.) The wort is allowed to settle so that the protein, which clouds beer, can be removed; the clear liquid is then fermented with yeast and aged. Eventually, yeast residue is skimmed off and used as a nutritional supplement (brewer's yeast) or added to livestock feed. The process may be varied and other ingredients added to give beer a distinctive flavor, color, or aroma. Adding extra hops produces the British draft beer known as bitters; ale, a more concentrated beer, uses a type of yeast that rises to the top; stout is a bitter ale brewed from a dark malt.

The specific brewing method influences the nutritional quality of beer. The cloudy German *weisse bier,* for example, retains many of the B vitamins

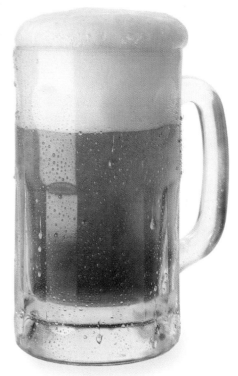

found in brewer's yeast, but these are strained away to make clear beer. Native African beers remain unfiltered; as a result, they retain many of the nutrients found in the grains and roots and tubers that are their main ingredients. The type of yeast used by Canadian brewers contains selenium, an antioxidant mineral, and chromium, a mineral that aids carbohydrate metabolism.

Nevertheless, the nutritional value of beer is often overstated because most of the nutrients in grain are lost in the brewing process. About two-thirds of the 150 calories in 12 ounces of ordinary beer come from the alcohol itself, with one-third coming from sugars; in contrast, only a trace of protein remains after brewing and straining. A 12-ounce bottle of ordinary beer provides 10 percent or more of the RNIs of folate, niacin, vitamin B_6, phosphorus, and magnesium as well as significant amounts of chromium and selenium.

HOW MUCH IS ENOUGH?

Typically, the alcohol content of beer ranges from 3 to 8 percent, compared to an average of 12 percent in wine and about 40 to 50 percent in hard liquor. Some people who are very sensitive to alcohol will react almost immediately to even this modest amount, often with feelings of aggression. Many people, however, can consume a quart or more of beer without obvious mental or physical effects. Since drinking more than a quart of fluid produces an uncomfortable feeling of fullness, most beer drinkers usually stop before they become inebriated. Even so, drinking a quart of beer may yield up to 600 calories, which can result in weight gain, and the excessive urination resulting from the diuretic effect of the alcohol can wash away important vitamins and minerals before the body can absorb them. Contrary to popular belief, chronic overconsumption of beer can lead to problem drinking and alcoholism.

Beer is frequently served with nuts, potato chips, pretzels, and other salty foods. Because these increase feelings of thirst, they actually promote consumption of excessive amounts of beer. Foods that are high in protein, starches, vitamins, and minerals are better alternatives to balance the high-sugar content of beer; for example, eggs, meat, poultry, seafood, or such starchy foods as whole-grain bread or crackers, pasta, and legumes.

BEETS

BENEFITS
- *A good source of folate and vitamin C.*
- *The greens are a rich source of potassium, calcium, iron, beta carotene, and vitamin C.*
- *Low in calories.*

DRAWBACKS
- *Turn urine and stools red, a harmless condition that nonetheless alarms people who mistake it for blood.*

Beets are a highly versatile vegetable. They can be boiled and served as a side dish, pickled and eaten as a salad or condiment, or used as the main ingredient in borscht, a popular Eastern European cold summer soup. Beet greens, the most nutritious part of the vegetable, can be cooked and served like spinach or Swiss chard.

According to folklore, beets were believed to possess curative powers for headaches and other painful conditions. Even today, some naturalist practitioners recommend beets to prevent cancer and bolster immunity; they also suggest using the juice of raw beets to speed convalescence. Although beets are a reasonably nutritious food source, there is no scientific proof that they confer any special medicinal benefits.

A half-cup serving of beets provides 45mcg (micrograms) of folate, about

one-fourth the adult Recommended Nutrient Intake (RNI), and 5mg of vitamin C. The tops, if eaten while young and green, are more nutritious: 1 cup supplies 35mg of vitamin C, almost 90 percent of the RNI for adults; 720 RE of Vitamin A; and 160mg of calcium, 2.5mg of iron, and 1,300mg of potassium.

The most flavorful beets are small, with greens still attached. The best way to cook beet roots is to boil them unpeeled, which retains most of the nutrients as well as the deep red color. After the beets have cooled, the skins slip off easily; the root can be sliced, chopped, or puréed, depending upon the method of serving. Beets may also be canned and pickled with vinegar; some nutrients are lost in the processing, but the sweet beet flavor remains.

EFFECTS ON BODY WASTES

Many people become alarmed when they notice that their urine and stools have turned pink or even red after eating beets. This is a harmless condition that occurs in about 15 percent of people who lack the gut bacteria that normally degrade betalains, the bright red pigment in beets. The urine and stools usually return to their normal colors after a day or two.

BEGINNER FOODS—FEEDING A BABY

Proper early nutrition is extremely important. The eating patterns established in infancy not only determine how well a baby grows but also influence lifelong food habits and attitudes.

New parents probably worry more about feeding their baby than any other aspect of early child care. What if I can't breast-feed? How do I know if the baby is getting enough? Too much? Should I give the baby vitamins? When do I start solid food? Parents quickly learn that almost everyone is eager to answer such questions—grandparents, doctors, nurses, neighbors, babysitters, casual acquaintances—even strangers in the supermarket. As might be expected, however, much of the advice is conflicting and adds to a parent's feelings of confusion and uncertainty. So let's begin with some general guidelines that should help ease some of the anxiety associated with feeding an infant:

First, get to know your baby. No two infants are alike. Some enter the world ravenously hungry and demand to be fed every hour or two. Others seem to prefer sleeping, and may even need to be awakened to eat.

Second, try to relax and enjoy your baby. It's natural for new parents to feel nervous and apprehensive, not sure if they are doing everything the right way, but raising a baby should be a joyful experience.

Third, learn to trust your own judgment and common sense. If a baby is growing and developing at a normal pace, he's getting enough to eat. With a little practice, you'll learn how to adjust the diet to the baby's needs.

Finally, keep food in its proper perspective. It provides the essential energy and nourishment infants need to grow and develop. But food should not be a substitute for a reassuring hug or used as a bribe or reward for good behavior. If parents respond accordingly, even an

FIRST MOUTHFULS. *Family mealtimes around the table give a newly weaned infant the opportunity to experience a variety of new tastes and food textures.*

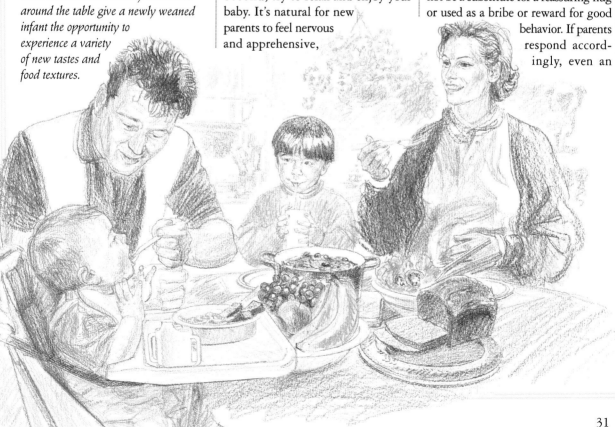

infant quickly learns how to use food as a manipulative tool, which can set the stage for later eating problems.

IN THE BEGINNING

Good infant nutrition actually begins before birth, because what the mother eats during pregnancy goes a long way toward determining her baby's nutritional needs. Skimping on food to avoid gaining excessive weight while pregnant can produce a low-birth-weight baby who not only has special nutritional needs but may also have serious medical problems. An anemic woman is likely to have a baby with low iron reserves. A woman who does not consume adequate folate may have a baby with serious neurological problems. Conversely, high doses of vitamin A just before and during early pregnancy can cause birth defects. Because of these potential problems, all pregnant women are strongly advised to have regular prenatal checkups and to eat a varied and balanced diet.

Physicians are in agreement that breast milk provides the best and most complete nutrition for full-term infants. (Premature and low-birth-weight babies may need special supplements.) Even if the mother plans to bottle-feed later, her baby benefits from just a few breast-feedings. Colostrum, the breast fluid that is secreted for the first few days after birth, is higher in protein and lower in sugar and fat than later breast milk. It has a laxative effect that activates the baby's bowels. Colostrum is also rich in antibodies, which increase the baby's resistance to infection.

Hormones released in response to the baby's suckling increase the flow of breast milk, and within a few days most women produce more than enough milk for their infants. This milk is easy to digest and provides just about all the nutrients that a baby normally needs for the first 4 to 6 months; however, many pediatricians recommend fluoride and vitamin D supplements beginning in the third or fourth month. In the past, iron supplements were given because breast milk contains very little of this mineral. Many doctors now feel that these are unnecessary; full-term babies born to women who are not anemic have enough iron reserves to last until they begin eating iron-fortified cereals and other foods (see Introducing New Foods in the First Year, p.35).

Many new nursing mothers often worry that their babies are not getting enough to eat. A baby who has regular stools and produces six or more wet diapers a day is most likely getting plenty of food. Although this varies

THE ADVANTAGES OF BREAST-FEEDING

• In the early postpartum period, nursing stimulates uterine contractions that help prevent hemorrhaging and return the uterus to its normal size. Breast-feeding also helps a woman lose the extra weight gained during pregnancy.

• Breast milk is more convenient and economical than formula; it is sterile, portable, and always the right temperature.

• Nursing promotes a special kind of mother-infant bonding and closeness.

• Breast-fed babies have a reduced incidence of bacterial meningitis and respiratory and intestinal disorders. The benefits appear to extend beyond childhood; recent studies show that people who were breast-fed have a reduced incidence of allergies, obesity, diabetes, inflammatory bowel disease, asthma and other chronic lung disorders, heart disease, and some types of cancer.

• Women who breast-feed appear to have a reduced risk of premenopausal breast cancer and postmenopausal osteoporosis (loss of bone mass).

considerably, breast-fed babies generally nurse every 2 to 4 hours for the first month or so. At one time, doctors felt that babies should be fed according to a regular schedule rather than on demand. This approach to nursing has fallen out of favor, and experts now agree that babies should be fed whenever they are hungry for the first 4 or 5 months. Some babies, however, may be overly sleepy or disinterested in food; a baby who is not feeding at least six to eight times a day may need to be awakened and stimulated to consume more.

Of course, growth is another important indicator of whether or not a baby is getting enough to eat. Remember, however, that babies and young children tend to grow in spurts, rather than showing a steady gain of a few ounces a week. During a growth spurt, an infant will want to nurse more often and longer than usual, which may completely empty the breasts. This will signal the mother's body to increase milk production. But the mother should not be concerned if, a week or two later, her baby is less interested in eating.

BOTTLE-FEEDING

Although more than half of all Canadian women now breast-feed for at least the first few weeks, this still leaves many who, for various reasons, elect to bottle-feed. They should be assured that commercial infant formulas provide all the essential nutrients and, when used according to the manufacturers' instructions, babies thrive on them. Babies under one year of age should not be given regular cow's milk because it is difficult for them to digest and it also may provoke an allergic reaction. The cow's milk in most infant formulas is modified to make it easier to digest. Despite this precaution, some babies are unable to tolerate it; these infants can usually digest a soy or rice formula.

Generally, bottle-fed babies consume more at a feeding than breast-fed infants do; they may also gain weight more rapidly, although the breast-fed babies will eventually catch up with them. On average, most babies double their birth weight in 4 to 5 months, and triple it by the time of their first birthday.

Bottle-feeding requires more work than nursing; bottles, nipples, and other equipment must be sterilized. Some formulas are premixed and can be used straight from the can; others are concentrated or powdered, and must be mixed with sterile water. Formula mixed in advance should be refrigerated, but not for any longer than 24 hours; after that, the formula should be discarded. Any formula that is left in the baby's bottle after a feeding also should be thrown away; if not, there is a possibility of its being contaminated by microorganisms entering through the nipple opening.

INTRODUCING FOODS

There is no specific age at which solid foods should be started, but for most babies, 4 or 5 months is about right. Starting too early can be harmful because the digestive system may not be able to handle solid foods yet; also, the early introduction of solid foods seems to increase the risk of developing food allergies. An infant who is thriving solely on breast milk can generally wait until he is 5 or even 6 months old; after that, however, nursing alone will not provide adequate calories and the range of nutrients that a baby needs for normal growth.

There are several typical signs that indicate when a baby is ready to move on to solid foods: The baby chews at the nipple instead of simply suckling it; he swallows food instead of spitting it out because of improved coordination of the tongue and mouth muscles; and he drools more, which will facilitate swallowing.

Case Study

When Jason was born, his mother elected to breast-feed him, at least for the first few months. Jason seemed to be thriving, but every now and then he developed diarrhea and was unusually fussy. When the pediatrician examined Jason, she found him to be a healthy baby with no abnormalities that would explain the diarrhea and excessive fussiness.

The doctor's next step was to question Martha, Jason's mother, about her diet and habits, explaining that many substances in foods, drinks, and medications find their way into breast milk. Martha couldn't pinpoint anything that might be causing Jason's problems, so the doctor asked her to keep a food diary, and also to note any accompanying symptoms in Jason.

After a week, the problem became clear. Whenever Martha ate onions and garlic—common ingredients in many of her favorite dishes—Jason responded with diarrhea and fussiness.

Martha then tried a week of abstaining from onions and garlic, and Jason was his usual cheerful self with absolutely normal stools. This was enough to convince Martha to forgo onions and garlic until after Jason was weaned—a small price to pay for a happy, comfortable baby.

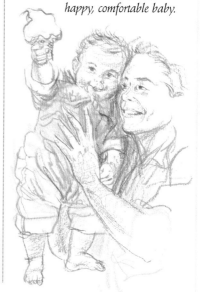

The first solid foods must be easy to digest and unlikely to provoke an allergic reaction—from both perspectives, infant rice cereal is a good choice. It can be mixed with formula, breast milk, or sterile water and fed with a spoon. For the first few feedings, put a very small amount of the cereal on the spoon, gently touch the baby's lips to encourage him to open his mouth, and try to place the cereal at the back of the tongue. Don't expect these feedings to go smoothly; even a baby who is ready for solid foods usually does a lot of spitting, sputtering, and protesting.

The baby should be hungry, but not ravenous. Some experts suggest starting the feeding with a few minutes of nursing or bottle-feeding, then offering a small amount of the moistened cereal—no more than a teaspoon or two—and finishing with the milk. After a few sessions, you can start with the cereal, then gradually increase the amount of solid foods at each feeding as you eventually reduce the amount of nursing or bottle-feeding.

Go slow in the beginning, introducing only one or two new items a week. If you use home-cooked foods, make sure that they're thoroughly puréed. In addition to iron-fortified rice cereal, try oatmeal and barley cereals; strained peas, carrots, sweet potatoes, and squash; applesauce, strained peaches and pears, and mashed bananas; and puréed chicken, turkey, lamb, and beef. Introduce vegetables before fruits, otherwise the baby may become hooked on the sweeter-tasting foods and reject the vegetables. If the baby refuses a particular food, don't force the issue; it's better to substitute something else and try again in a few weeks.

At about 5 months, fruit juice can be added to the diet, starting with apple juice. Hold off on orange juice and other citrus products for at least 6 months; these may provoke an allergic reaction. Other potentially allergenic foods should be delayed until the baby is 6 to 9 months old, or even later if there is a family history of allergies; such foods include corn, wheat products, berries, fish, and spinach. It's best to wait until after the first birthday to give the baby egg whites—one of the most allergenic foods—although the yolks can be tried somewhat earlier. Withdraw any food that provokes a rash, runny nose, unusual fussiness, diarrhea, or any other sign of a possible allergic reaction or food intolerance.

SELF-FEEDING

When they are about 7 or 8 months old, most babies have developed enough eye-hand coordination to pick up finger food and maneuver it into their mouths. The teeth are also beginning to erupt at this age; giving a baby an unsalted pretzel, teething biscuit, or cracker to chew on can ease gum soreness as well as provide practice in self-feeding. Other good starter finger foods include bite-size dry cereals, bananas, slices of apples and pears, peas, and cooked carrots, and small pieces of soft-cooked boiled or roasted chicken, ground beef, and turkey. The pieces should be large enough to hold but small enough so that they don't lodge in the throat and cause choking. For this reason, foods like grapes and peanuts should be avoided until the child is older.

As soon as the baby can sit in a high chair, he should be included in at least some family meals and start eating many of the same foods, even though they may need mashing or cutting into small pieces. Give the child a spoon, but don't be disappointed if he

prefers using his hands. Try not to be too concerned about spills, which are inevitable; you can spread a plastic sheet on the floor to facilitate cleaning up (it should probably extend well beyond the high chair). At this stage it's more important for the baby to become integrated into family activities and master self-feeding than to learn neatness and proper table manners. These will come eventually, especially if the parents and older siblings set a good example.

WEANING

Giving up the breast or bottle is a major milestone in a baby's development, but not one that should be rushed. When a woman stops nursing is largely a matter of personal preference. Some mothers wean their babies from the breast to a bottle after only a few weeks or months; others continue nursing for 18 months or longer, even though the child is eating solid food and perhaps drinking milk from a cup. Similarly, some babies decide to give up their bottles themselves at 9 or 10 months; yet others will still want it—especially at nap or bedtime—until they are 2 years old or even older. In any event, a baby should

not be given regular cow's milk in the first year of life. If a baby under a year old drinks milk from a cup, it should still be a formula.

DENTAL HYGIENE

Many parents mistakenly assume that baby, or primary, teeth aren't important because they are eventually replaced by permanent teeth. In fact, early dental decay not only threatens the underlying secondary teeth, it can cause severe toothaches. As soon as the first tooth erupts, parents should begin practicing preventive dental hygiene. Babies should not be permitted to fall asleep while nursing or sucking a bottle; this allows milk to pool in the mouth, and the sugar (lactose) in it can cause extensive tooth decay. Offering a little water at the end of a feeding rinses any remaining milk from the baby's mouth. The gums and emerging teeth can be wiped gently with a gauze-wrapped finger.

Sugar is the major cause of childhood tooth decay; avoid offering sugary soft drinks and sweet snacks. Fruit juice, boiled water, a chunk of cheese, or a piece of fruit are better alternatives that provide important nutrients without harming the teeth.

COMMERCIAL BABY FOODS

Most babies' introduction to solid food comes in the form of small jars of puréed vegetables, fruits, and meats. Older babies graduate to thicker and chunkier commercial foods prepared for toddlers. For a young baby, the commercial foods offer several advantages. They are safe, and most are now salt- and sugar-free. For the mother, they offer convenience. But they also have disadvantages. They are expensive, they offer the baby little incentive to develop chewing and self-feeding skills, and they have

less nutritional value than freshly prepared foods. If you do elect to use commercial baby foods, follow these precautions:
• Never feed the baby straight from the jar and then save the remaining food; saliva on the spoon can transmit bacteria to the food and result in spoilage.
• Commercial baby food tastes bland; resist the temptation to season it with salt. Excessive salt can cause later health problems, especially if there is a family history of high blood pressure.

Introducing New Foods in the First Year

During the first 3 months of life, breast milk or formula provides all the nutrients a newborn baby needs. The following chart summarizes the generally accepted guidelines for introducing new foods to babies under a year old. It should be noted, however, that all babies are different; consequently, the timing varies considerably from one baby to another.

1 to 3 MONTHS Total intake: About 2½ oz of formula or breast milk per pound of body weight.

First month: If giving breast milk, enough for weight gain and to yield regular soft stools and at least 6–8 wet diapers a day. If giving formula, 2–4 oz per feeding (every 2 to 4 hours).

Second and third months: 4–5 oz each feeding; six feedings a day.

MILK AND DAIRY	CEREALS AND OTHER STARCHY FOODS	VEGETABLES AND FRUITS	MEAT AND MEAT ALTERNATIVES	OCCASIONAL FOODS
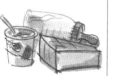	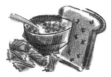	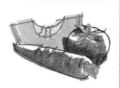	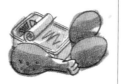	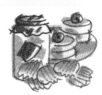

4 to 6 MONTHS Total intake: About 30 oz per day of breast milk or formula, plus small amounts (1 or 2 teaspoons) of new foods (introduced one at a time) at two or three feedings a day.

MILK AND DAIRY	CEREALS AND OTHER STARCHY FOODS	VEGETABLES AND FRUITS	MEAT AND MEAT ALTERNATIVES	OCCASIONAL FOODS
By 4 months: 5–6 oz breast milk or formula each feeding five or six times a day.	**At 4 months:** Start with rice cereal, followed by oatmeal and barley. Begin with ½ teaspoonful or less; then gradually work up to 1 or 2 teaspoonfuls.	**At 4 to 5 months:** Start with small amounts of puréed vegetables (peas, carrots, squash, etc.); after a few weeks, add strained or puréed fruits (applesauce, bananas, peaches, pears, etc.).	**At 5 to 6 months:** Strained meats are usually one of the last foods to be added. The meat should be soft-cooked and puréed.	Babies tend to like bland foods, so salt is not needed. Salty or sugary drinks and snacks should be avoided; use boiled water instead. Small amounts of apple juice can be added at 5 to 6 months.

7 to 8 MONTHS Total intake: By the end of 6 months, about 30–40 oz of breast milk or formula; 2–4 oz. of cereal and/or puréed baby food should be given at each of the baby's three meals.

MILK AND DAIRY	CEREALS AND OTHER STARCHY FOODS	VEGETABLES AND FRUITS	MEAT AND MEAT ALTERNATIVES	OCCASIONAL FOODS
For breast milk, continue or wean to bottle. Give five or six feedings per day. For formula, 6–8 oz per feeding four or five times each day.	Other breads and cereals may be added, but avoid wheat products. Begin serving finger foods, such as dry toast squares or bite-size cereals. **Daily intake:** ¼ to ½ cup of starchy food over three meals.	Increase the variety of fruits and vegetables, but avoid corn, berries, citrus fruits, and spinach. **Daily intake:** Four ¼- to ½-cup servings of noncitrus juices, fruits, and vegetables.	Softened meat can be cut up into small pieces to be eaten as finger food. **Daily intake:** Two ½- to ¾-oz portions of meat, cheese, or other meat alternatives.	Citrus fruit juices tend to irritate the baby's skin and make stools acidic, so it is advisable to wait until at least 6 to 9 months.

9 to 12 MONTHS 750 to 900 total calories needed per day divided into three meals and two snacks.

MILK AND DAIRY	CEREALS AND OTHER STARCHY FOODS	VEGETABLES AND FRUITS	MEAT AND MEAT ALTERNATIVES	OCCASIONAL FOODS
Add yogurt and milk puddings. **Daily intake:** About 24 oz breast milk or formula per day (400–500 calories).	Wheat and mixed cereals may be added, as well as other starches, such as potatoes, rice, and well-cooked pasta. **Daily intake:** ½- to ¾-cup total a day.	A mixture of fruits (including juices) and vegetables distributed during meals and snacks. **Daily intake:** Six ¼-cup servings a day.	Egg yolks may be tried, but avoid whites until after the first birthday. Egg whites may cause an allergic reaction. **Daily intake:** Total of 2 oz of meat a day.	May use moderate amounts of butter (unsalted) and small amounts of jam on bread, toast, and crackers. Do not give peanut butter, which can cause choking.

CANCER

EAT PLENTY OF
- *Citrus and other fruits and dark green or yellow vegetables for vitamin C, beta carotene, bioflavonoids, and other plant chemicals that protect against cancer.*
- *Whole-grain breads and cereals and other high-fiber foods to promote smooth colon function.*

CUT DOWN ON
- *Fatty foods, especially those high in saturated animal fats.*
- *Alcoholic beverages.*
- *Salt-cured, smoked, fermented, and charcoal-broiled foods.*

AVOID
- *Foods that may contain pesticide residues and environmental pollutants.*

Recent research has dramatically changed our thinking about the role of diet in both the prevention and treatment of cancer. It's increasingly clear that certain dietary elements may help promote the development and spread of malignancies, while others slow or block tumor growth. The Canadian Cancer Society estimates that one out of three cancers may be related to diet, especially one high in fat and processed foods; they also believe that most of these cancers could be prevented by dietary changes.

PROTECTIVE FOODS

Compelling data associate a diet that provides ample fruits and vegetables with a reduced risk of many of our most deadly cancers. These foods are rich in bioflavonoids and other plant chemicals; dietary fiber; and ANTIOXIDANTS, vitamins A, C, and E, and selenium. All of these substances may slow, stop, or reverse the processes that can lead to cancer. They do so through several protective mechanisms: by neutralizing or detoxifying cancer-causing agents (car-cinogens); by preventing precancerous changes in cellular genetic material due to carcinogens, radiation, and other environmental factors; by inducing the formation of protective enzymes; and by reducing the hormonal action that can stimulate tumor growth.

Equally important is a reduced intake of FATS. Numerous studies link a high-fat diet and obesity with an increased risk of cancers of the colon, uterus, prostate, and skin (including melanoma, the most deadly form of skin cancer). The link between fat consumption and breast cancer is more controversial. Experts stress that no more than 30 percent of total calories should come from fats, and many feel that even this is too high, advocating a 20 percent limit on fat calories. Often, it takes only a few simple dietary changes to lower fat intake; for example, choosing lean cuts of meat, trimming away all visible fat, substituting pasta and other vegetarian dishes for meat several times a week, adopting low-fat cooking methods, such as baking and steaming, and limiting the use of butter, margarine, mayonnaise, shortening, and oils.

Increased intake of fiber may protect against cancer in several ways. It speeds the transit of waste through the colon, which some researchers think cuts the risk of bowel cancer. A high-fiber, low-calorie diet also protects against obesity and the increased risk of cancers linked to excessive body fat.

HARMFUL HABITS

Doctors warn against heavy use of alcohol, which is associated with an increased risk of cancers of the mouth, larynx, esophagus, and liver. Excessive alcohol consumption hinders the body's ability to use beta carotene, which appears to protect against these cancers. Alcohol can also deplete reserves of folate, thiamine, and other B vitamins, as well as selenium. Folate is known to re-

> ## EAT YOUR VEGETABLES (AND FRUITS TOO)!
>
> The pigments and other chemicals that give plant foods their bright colors also seem to contribute to their cancer-fighting properties. Nutritionists now agree with the age-old urging of mothers and advise people to eat at least three different-colored vegetables and two different fruits daily. Choose from among the dark green leafy vegetables and the dark yellow, orange, and red fruits and vegetables. Include one serving of citrus a day, and strive to have a cruciferous vegetable. The members of the cruciferous (or cabbage) family include bok choy, broccoli, Brussels sprouts, cabbage, cauliflower, collards, kale, kohlrabi, mustard greens, rutabagas, and turnips.

duce proliferation of cancer cells; low levels of folate are also associated with an increased risk of cervical cancer. Researchers have found that giving folate supplements slows the proliferation of other precancerous cells.

Smoking, more than any other lifestyle factor, increases the risk of cancer; stopping the habit is the most important step that a smoker can take to avoid cancer. In addition to lung cancer, smoking is strongly associated with cancers of the esophagus, mouth, larynx, pancreas, and bladder; recent studies also link it to an increased risk of breast cancer. For people who find it impossible to stop smoking, there are a few dietary measures that can somewhat lower their cancer risk. One is to consume broccoli or related cruciferous vegetables several times a week. These members of the cabbage family are known to be appreciably high in certain cancer-fighting compounds, including bioflavonoids, indoles, monoterpenes, phenolic acids, and plant sterols, precursors to vitamin D. In addition, sulforaphane, a chemical particularly abundant in broccoli, is one of the most potent anticancer compounds identified to date; various studies show that eating broccoli several times a week lowers the incidence of lung cancer among smokers compared to those whose diet does not include the vegetable.

Low levels of vitamin C are linked to an increased risk of many of the cancers related to smoking. Because smoking works to deplete the body's reserves of vitamin C, it's a good idea for smokers to increase their intake of citrus fruits and other good sources of this nutrient. Similarly, smoking can deplete the body's stores of folate and other B complex vitamins; increased consumption of lean meat, grains, fortified cereals, legumes, and green leafy vegetables may help counter this adverse effect.

People who eat large amounts of smoked, pickled, cured, fried, charcoal-broiled, and processed meats have a

high incidence of stomach and esophageal tumors. Smoked foods contain polyaromatic hydrocarbons which are known carcinogens. The salt in pickled foods can injure the stomach wall and facilitate tumor formation. Nitrites and nitrates in processed meats can form nitrosamines, established carcinogens. However, consuming these foods along with good sources of vitamins C and E reduces the formation of nitrosamines.

WHEN CANCER STRIKES

A qualified nutritionist should be part of any cancer treatment team, because both the disease and its treatment demand good nutrition as an aid to recovery. Surgery, which still remains the major treatment for cancer, also requires a highly nutritious diet for healing and recuperation. The cancer itself can cause nutritional problems that will require treatment along with the underlying disease; for example, colon cancer will often cause iron-deficiency ANEMIA because of chronic intestinal bleeding.

Weight loss is common among almost all cancer patients. Most experience anorexia, or loss of appetite, as a result of the cancer itself; depression brought on by a diagnosis of a potentially fatal disease, as well as pain, understandably lessens any desire to eat. Cancer treatments, especially radiation and chemotherapy, curb appetite and produce nausea and other side effects. Surgery, too, can affect appetite and make eating undesirable, especially if it involves the digestive system. A dietitian or qualified nutritionist can devise a diet or recommend supplements to provide the calories, protein, and other nutrients needed to maintain weight and promote healing.

Dietary guidelines for cancer patients must take into account the stage and type of malignancy. In most cases of early or localized cancer, patients are generally advised to follow a diet that is low in fat; high in pasta, whole-grain products, and other starches; and high in fruits and vegetables. Fats, especially from animal sources, are discouraged because they are believed to support tumor growth. In contrast, fruits and vegetables contain an assortment of natural plant chemicals that are thought to retard cancer growth and spread.

Protein and zinc are essential for wound healing; therefore, surgery patients should eat two or more daily servings of lean meat, low-fat milk, eggs, fish, and shellfish. Many cancer patients find it difficult to tolerate red meat, however, because it takes on an unpleasant metallic taste; in such instances, substituting egg whites, poultry, and a combination of

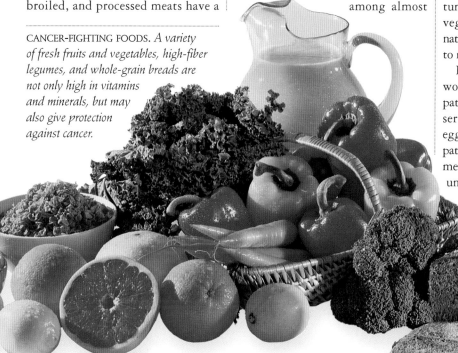

CANCER-FIGHTING FOODS. *A variety of fresh fruits and vegetables, high-fiber legumes, and whole-grain breads are not only high in vitamins and minerals, but may also give protection against cancer.*

COPING WITH EATING PROBLEMS

In many instances, loss of appetite, nausea, and other eating problems of cancer patients can be dealt with by changing daily habits and routines. The following tips have worked for many people.

• Plan your major meal for the time of day when you are least likely to experience nausea and vomiting. For many cancer patients, this is in the early morning. Otherwise, eat small, frequent meals and snacks throughout the day.

• Let someone else prepare the food; cooking odors often provoke nausea. Food that is served cold or at room temperature gives off less odor than hot food.

• If mouth sores are a problem, eat bland, puréed foods—for example, custards, rice and other puddings made with milk and eggs, porridge, and blended soups. Avoid salty, spicy, or acidic foods. Sucking on zinc lozenges may speed the healing of mouth sores.

• Try to eat with others in a pleasant social atmosphere. Ask family members to bring home-cooked food to the hospital (but have them check with the dietitian first).

• Get dressed to eat, if possible, and strive to make meals visually attractive. A few slices of a colorful fruit give visual appeal to a bowl of oatmeal; a colorful napkin and bud vase perk up a tray of food.

• To overcome nausea, try chewing on ice chips or sucking on a ginger candy or sour lemon drop before eating. Sipping flat ginger ale or cola may also help.

• Rest for half an hour after eating, preferably in a sitting or upright position; reclining may trigger reflux, nausea, and vomiting.

• Pay extra attention to dental hygiene. If mouth sores hinder tooth brushing, make a baking soda paste and use your finger and a soft cloth to gently cleanse the teeth. Then rinse the mouth with a weak solution of hydrogen peroxide and baking soda. Diluted commercial mouth washes freshen the breath, but avoid full-strength products that can further irritate sores.

• If a dry mouth makes swallowing difficult, liquefy foods in a blender or moisten them with low-fat milk, sauces, or gravies.

• If diarrhea is a problem (as is often the case during chemotherapy), avoid fatty foods, raw fruits, whole-grain products, and other foods that can make it worse. Instead, eat bland, binding foods, such as rice, bananas, cooked apples, and dry toast.

---

legumes and grains will provide the needed protein and zinc. In some cases, supplements may be prescribed.

WISDOM OF THE BODY

Flying in the face of conventional wisdom, however, are recent recommendations from a growing number of cancer specialists who discourage urging some cancer patients to eat when they don't feel like it. In the past, forced feeding in the form of enriched dietary supplements, intravenous nutrition, or a gastric feeding tube was recommended to maintain nutrition, but these approaches usually did not result in weight gain or prolonged survival. Instead, many who were force-fed actually died sooner; experts now believe this may be because the feeding actually spurs tumor growth. Consequently, many medical scientists now believe that the anorexia and cachexia (a severe form of malnutrition and body wasting) that occurs in advanced cancer may be an example of the "wisdom of the body" as it attempts to starve the tumor. Although it may be difficult for family members and friends to watch loved ones stop eating and progressively lose weight, informed physicians now urge that, in some situations, cachectic patients be allowed to limit food intake while doctors undertake aggressive therapy to destroy the tumor. Once this is accomplished, appetite returns, and the lost weight is regained as recovery takes place.

THE LURE OF SUPPLEMENTS

Millions of North Americans take vitamin and mineral supplements, often in high doses and without consulting a doctor. Recent reports detailing the anticancer effects of antioxidants have resulted in greatly increased sales of high-dose supplements of beta carotene and vitamins A, C, and E. In theory, it is reasonable to assume that if a small amount of a nutrient protects against cancer, then a high dose should be even more protective. Unfortunately, this does not seem to be true. When consumed in the amounts that are generally found in foods, these nutrients do have an antioxidant effect, which prevents the potentially cancer-causing damage that occurs when the body uses oxygen. But when taken in the form of high-dose supplements, these substances may have an opposite effect; recent research indicates they may become pro-oxidants and may actually increase damage caused by free radicals, the unstable molecules released when the body uses oxygen. In addition, high doses of vitamin A can lead to toxicity.

The situation may be quite different, however, for patients who are undergoing cancer treatment. Some may need high-dose supplements, while others may be advised to avoid certain nutrients. This is why it's important to consult a registered dietitian or nutritionist regarding any dietary change and supplementation. There is no scientific evidence to suggest that alternative therapies, which include Japanese maitake, Chinese herbs, blue-green algae, and shark cartilage extracts, have any value in cancer treatment.

CARBOHYDRATES: THE BACKBONE OF A HEALTHY DIET

Starches and sugars are our major source of energy.
In their natural state, they are also low in
calories and high in fiber, vitamins, and minerals.

Almost all of the starches and sugars that humans burn for energy come from plants; the only major exception is lactose, the sugar in milk. In effect, each plant is a complex food factory that takes water from the soil, carbon dioxide from the air, and energy from the sun to make glucose, a simple sugar that is later converted into starch. As the plant develops and grows, it also makes various vitamins, minerals, and chemicals, as well as some fat and protein. Consequently, we can get our carbohydrates and most of the other nutrients needed to sustain life from thousands of different grains, seeds, fruits, and vegetables.

In general, carbohydrates are classified according to their chemical structure and digestibility; they are divided into two groups:

Simple carbohydrates, or sugars, form crystals that dissolve in water and are easily digested. Naturally occurring sugars occur in a variety of fruits, some vegetables, honey, and maple sap. Processed sugars include table sugar, brown sugar, and molasses.

Complex carbohydrates have a range of textures, flavors, colors, and molecular structures. Composed of complex chains of sugars, these carbohydrates are further classified as starches and fiber. Our digestive system can break down and metabolize most starches, which are found in an array of grains, vegetables, and some fruits. The digestive system lacks the enzymes or or-

---

> **BENEFITS**
> - *They are converted to glucose, which the body uses for energy.*
> - *Starchy foods are low in cost, yet high in nutritional value.*
>
> **DRAWBACKS**
> - *Simple carbohydrates (various sugars) are low in nutritional value; in addition, they usually promote dental decay.*

---

ganisms that are needed to break down most fiber, including cellulose and other woody parts of the plant skeleton, and pectin and other gums that hold plant cells together. But dietary fiber is still important because it promotes smooth colon function and may help prevent some types of cancer, heart attacks, and other diseases.

HOW CARBOHYDRATES WORK

Our body metabolizes both simple and complex carbohydrates into glucose, or blood sugar, the body's primary source of fuel. Carbohydrates are high-quality fuels because—compared to proteins or fats—relatively little work is required of the body to break them down in order to release their energy.

Glucose, the only form of carbohydrates that the body can use immediately, is essential for the functioning of the brain, nervous system, muscles, and various organs. At any given time the blood can carry about an hour's supply of glucose. Any glucose that is not needed for immediate energy is converted into glycogen and stored in the liver and muscles; when it is required, the liver turns the glycogen back into glucose. The body can store only enough glycogen to last for several hours of moderate activity.

The glycemic index is a measure of how quickly the energy from a carbohydrate food is made available for use as glucose, as reflected by the raising of the blood sugar level. Sugars are rapidly converted into glucose to provide energy. In contrast, starches vary widely in the glycemic response they generate, with the size of a food particle and the duration of cooking, if any, having a significant effect. The bigger the particle size, the more difficult it is to digest and the more slowly glucose is released into the bloodstream, yielding a lower "glycemic index." For example, stone-ground whole-grain bread has a larger particle size, and a lower glycemic index, than finely milled bread, whether white or whole-grain.

When glucose reserves run low, the body turns first to protein and then to fat to convert them into glucose. Burning protein, however, robs the body of lean muscle tissue. In addition, if the body has to burn fat in the absence of carbohydrates, toxic by-products called ketones are released; these can lead to a potentially dangerous biochemical imbalance.

THE IMPORTANCE OF STARCHES

Complex carbohydrates form the basis of the human diet worldwide. In Canada and many other industrialized countries, however, the bulk of calories comes from meat and other high-protein foods, fats, and simple carbohydrates (often in the form of processed sugars). Until recently, starchy foods have been shunned as being fattening, dull, and nutritionally unimportant. We now know that this is a serious misconception, which may account, at least in part, for our modern epidemics of obesity, diabetes, heart disease, and some types of CANCER.

Despite carbohydrates' undeserved reputation as being fattening, both carbohydrates and proteins provide 4 calories per gram, compared to 9 calories per gram of fat. Sugar and starches are fattening only when they are consumed with fatty additions or are eaten in quantities much larger than the body can readily use, in which case they are converted and stored as body fat. Overeating is unlikely to be a problem if meals are built around starchy and fibrous foods, which tend to be filling. In contrast, meat and other high-protein foods come pack-aged with fat and are more likely to cause weight gain.

Most grains, vegetables, and fruits also provide essential vitamins and minerals, making them even more important nutritionally. In contrast, pure sugars can be used for energy but offer no nutrients.

HOW MUCH DO YOU NEED?

The prevailing scientific wisdom is that approximately 55 to 60 percent of calories should come from carbohydrates drawn from a wide spectrum of grains and other starches, vegetables, and fruits. Only about 10 percent of these calories should be from processed sugars. Unfortunately, the typical North American diet now gets 20 percent of its calories from sugar, 20 percent from protein, 35 percent from fat, and only 25 percent from starches.

There are encouraging signs of improvement, however. Recent surveys show that an increasing number of people are eating more bread, cereals, pasta, grains, and legumes and are cutting back on meat. Although so-called refined carbohydrates, such as white flour and white rice, are just as good energy sources as whole-wheat flour and brown rice, processing removes many essential nutrients, including the B vitamins, iron and other minerals, and dietary fiber. The best approach is to build a diet around whole or lightly processed grains and raw or slightly cooked vegetables and fruits.

CARBOHYDRATE LOADING

Nutrition can have a significant impact on athletic performance and vice versa. Regular exercise increases the body's ability to utilize glucose efficiently and to store glycogen in muscle tissue. Thus, the fitter you are, the greater your ability to store the extra glycogen that is particularly needed for endurance events, such as running a marathon or cross-country skiing.

Therefore, although a well-balanced diet is important for anyone interested in complete nutrition, a diet high in carbohydrates is particularly beneficial for athletes. In general, nutritionists recommend that athletes who train exhaustively on a daily basis should aim for a diet with 65 to 70 percent of calories coming from carbohydrates. Further, 80 to 85 percent of these carbohydrates should come from starches, such as pasta, bread, cereals, grains, potatoes, and beans, with the balance coming from fruit and other sugary foods.

Athletes seeking to develop plentiful stores of glycogen have turned to "carbohydrate loading" before major athletic events. This involves consuming a diet that is very high in carbohydrates for 3 days, then really loading up the night before the event on a large meal of pasta, bread, and other starchy foods. This dietary strategy is useful in endurance sports or those that require an end burst of energy, such as competitive rowing.

SPECIAL CONCERNS

Carbohydrates can be incorporated into almost any diet, but people with certain diseases may need to

---

DID YOU KNOW?

• Carbohydrates make up about 75 percent of total calorie intake worldwide. In the developed world, however, they comprise only 45 percent of the diet, with almost half coming from sugars.

• Legumes, such as dried beans and peas, provide the best food value per dollar spent.

• Just because you don't see "sugar" listed as an ingredient on a food label doesn't mean it's not there. Look for words ending in "ose" (sucrose, lactose, maltose, fructose, glucose, and dextrose) and anything described as "syrup" (such as corn or malt syrup), as well as honey and molasses.

• Maltose is found in sprouting grains, malted wheat and barley, and malt extract.

• Glycogen is the form in which carbohydrates are stored in humans and animals, but it can be quickly converted back to glucose. Because it has a structure similar to starch, it is sometimes referred to as animal starch.

• After harvesting, the sugar in corn and other starchy vegetables is gradually converted to starch, which explains why these foods lose their sweetness. In contrast, the starch in bananas and other starchy fruits turns to sugar, increasing their sweetness.

CARBOHYDRATES IN THE DAILY DIET

Carbohydrates should provide about 55 to 60 percent of your total energy intake, with a balance of starchy foods, vegetables, and fruits. The Food Guide Rainbow (see p.23) recommends that a person with an energy need of 1,800 or more calories per day should eat 5 to 12 servings of starchy foods, 5 to 10 servings of fruits and vegetables. Below are three suggested combinations of carbohydrate foods that would fulfill the recommended number of servings for the average person. These are spread over the traditional three meals a day, but if desired, some can be switched to between-meal snacks. Follow Canada's Food Guide for recommendations to create your own combinations.

1 bowl cold whole-grain cereal
1 slice toast
½ grapefruit

2 slices whole-grain bread
1 large bowl of salad with lettuce,
  green pepper, cucumber, and tomato
1 apple

1 baked potato
½ cup broccoli
½ cup carrots
1 peach
2 oatmeal cookies

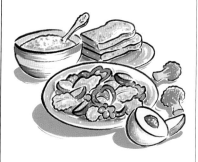

½ cup orange juice
1 bowl cooked whole-grain cereal
¼ cup raisins
1 muffin

Large three-bean salad (chickpeas, red
  kidney beans, and string beans)
½ cup rice
1 banana

Bowl of pasta with tomatoes, eggplant,
  peas, and tomato sauce
1 cup spinach salad
½ cup berries

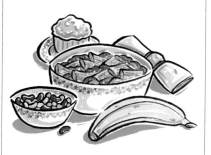

1 medium-size orange, sliced
2 slices French toast
½ cup applesauce

2 corn tortillas filled with beans,
  lettuce, tomato, and salsa
½ cup fruit salad
3-4 tea biscuits

1 sweet potato
½ cup lima beans
½ cup squash
½ cup pineapple
1 roll

make some adjustments. People with diabetes, for example, should include a balance of protein, fat, and high-fiber starchy foods, such as whole-grain bread, beans, peas, and lentils, at each meal. This balance provides for a steady supply of glucose, rather than the typical sharp rise that occurs after an all-carbohydrate meal. Contrary to popular belief, sugar does not cause diabetes, nor do diabetics have to completely avoid sugar. They do, however, have to monitor the blood level of glucose, but whether the glucose originates from table sugar or from starch is not relevant.

Sugar does contribute to dental disorders.

Those with heart disease need to emphasize high-fiber complex carbohydrates in their diet. Soluble FIBER, such as that found in oat bran and fruit pectin, helps lower high cholesterol levels and plays an important role in preventing atherosclerosis, the buildup of fatty deposits in coronary arteries and other blood vessels.

CANCER patients are often advised to increase their intake of carbohydrates and decrease fat intake, especially if they have cancers of the breast, colon, uterus, prostate, or skin. Increasing evidence suggests that fat in general, and animal fat in particular, may influence body chemistry in such a manner as to support tumor growth.

People with celiac disease should avoid all foods containing gluten, a protein found in wheat, rye, and to a lesser extent, other cereal grains. Because carbohydrates are easy to digest, they often make up the bulk of the diet for people with various digestive disorders. Depending on the nature of the disorder, high- or low-fiber foods may predominate.

CHILDHOOD AND ADOLESCENT NUTRITION

During the first few years of life, it's vital to meet a child's nutritional needs in order to ensure proper growth and also to establish a lifelong habit of healthy eating.

Eating a meal should be both a healthy and an enjoyable occasion—a fact that many parents may overlook when planning a meal for their growing children. Instead of a fast meal (especially one short in nutritional value) that family members eat at different hours, mealtimes should promote family togetherness.

Relaxed dining experiences with good food and conversation (that doesn't involve criticizing table manners or pleading with children to eat) help to foster family relationships as well as good digestion. You should try to schedule meals so that they don't conflict with other activities; children will be less likely to gobble their food and rush to leave the table. You can also involve children in family meals by having them help out with simple mealtime tasks, such as peeling potatoes, preparing salads, or setting the table. If mealtime is a pleasant event, children may practice healthful eating habits later on in life.

THE GROWING YEARS

Between the ages of 2 and 20, the human body changes continuously and dramatically. In general, muscles grow stronger, bones grow longer, height may more than double, and weight can increase as much as fivefold. The most striking changes take place during puberty, which usually occurs between the ages of 10 and 15 in girls and slightly later—between the ages of 12 and 19—in boys. Sexual development and maturity take place at this time, which, along with the adolescent growth spurt, result in a startling physical transformation.

Children need energy throughout the growing years: typically 1,300 calories a day for a 2-year-old, 1,700 for a 5-year-old, 2,200 for a 16-year-old girl, and 2,800 for a 16-year-old boy. For a guide to their nutritional needs, see Food for Growing Up, p.44.

The amount of food that a child needs

DO'S AND DON'TS: ENCOURAGING GOOD EATING HABITS

• Do set a good example for your child to copy. Share mealtimes and eat the same healthy foods.

• Do discourage snacking on sweets and fatty foods. Keep plenty of healthy foods, such as fruits, raw vegetables, low-fat crackers, and yogurt, around for children to eat between meals.

• Do allow children to follow their natural appetites when deciding how much to eat.

• Do encourage children to enjoy fruits and vegetables by giving them a variety from an early age.

• Don't give skim or 1-percent-fat milk to children under the age of 5 unless your doctor prescribes it; at this stage children need the extra calories in whole milk.

• Do ask children to help prepare meals. If parents rely mostly on convenience foods, children may not learn to enjoy cooking.

• Don't add unnecessary sugar to drinks and foods.

• Don't accustom children to extra salt by adding it to food or placing the shaker on the table.

• Don't give whole nuts to children under the age of 5, who may choke on them. Peanut butter and chopped nuts are fine as long as the child is not allergic to them.

• Don't force children to eat more than they want.

• Don't use food as a bribe.

• Don't make children feel guilty about eating any type of food.

varies according to height, build, gender, and activity level. Left to themselves, most children will usually eat the amount of food that's right for them; however, it is up to the parents to make sure that their children have the right foods available to choose from. Don't fall into the age-old trap of forcing them to eat more food than they want or need. Yesterday's notion of "cleaning your plate" and "starving children in Africa" can lead to overeating and weight problems or to a lifelong dislike of particular foods. Parents may find it better to serve smaller portions in the first place or to allow children to serve themselves.

CHANGES IN APPETITE

In most children, appetite slackens as the growth rate slows after the first year; it will then vary throughout childhood, depending on whether the child is going through a period of slow or rapid growth. It is perfectly normal for a young child to eat ravenously one day and then show little interest in food the following day.

Eating patterns change with the onset of the adolescent growth spurt; teenagers usually develop voracious appetites to match their need for additional energy. At the same time, many develop erratic eating habits— for example, skipping breakfast, lunching at school or at a fast-food restaurant, then snacking almost non-stop until bedtime. Although snacking is not the ideal way to eat, a "food on the run" lifestyle won't necessarily cause nutritional problems as long as the basic daily requirements for protein, carbohydrates, fats, and various vitamins and minerals are met. You can generally keep your teenager out of nutritional danger by providing snacks that are high in vitamins, minerals, and protein but low in sugar, fat, and salt. This basically means buying healthful snack foods, such as fresh and dried fruits, juices, raw vegetables, nuts, cheese, whole-grain crackers, unadulterated popcorn, and yogurt— not candy, cake, cookies, potato chips, corn chips, and soda pop.

THE QUESTION OF SWEETS

Sugary foods can provide a quick burst of energy, but they can also spoil the appetite for healthier foods and cause tooth decay without contributing any valuable nutrients. However, banning candies altogether can be troublesome; children may feel left out when their friends have them and so develop a pattern of eating candy in secret. There is no harm in letting children have candy occasionally, as long as you don't offer sweets as bribes or rewards for good behavior. For a sweet treat, cookies or ice cream is better than candy because there are some nutrients in the milk and grains used to make these snacks. If your family has dessert as a regular part of the menu,

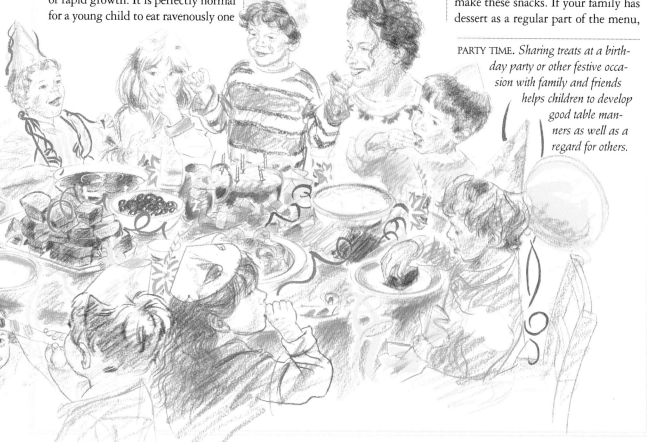

PARTY TIME. *Sharing treats at a birthday party or other festive occasion with family and friends helps children to develop good table manners as well as a regard for others.*

FOOD FOR GROWING UP

As children grow, their nutritional needs change; some needs vary between the sexes. The chart below gives an overview of the Recommended Nutrient Intakes (RNIs) of certain nutrients for children | *from ages 1 to 18. This information was compiled by the Nutrition Research Division of Health Canada. Height and weight estimates for each age group and sex are also included.*

AGE	1–3	4–6	7–10	11–14	15–18
HEIGHT (IN)	35	44	52	62	BOYS: 69 GIRLS: 64
WEIGHT (LB)	29	44	62	BOYS: 99 GIRLS: 101	BOYS: 145 GIRLS: 120
CALORIES Boys Girls	1,300 1,300	1,800 1,800	2,000 2,000	2,500 2,200	3,000 2,200
PROTEIN (G) Boys Girls	16 16	19 19	26 26	49 46	58 47
VITAMIN A (RE) Boys Girls	400 400	500 500	700 700	1,000 800	1,000 800
VITAMIN D (MCG)	10	5	2.5	2.5	2.5
VITAMIN E (MG) Boys Girls	4 4	5 5	7 7	10 8	10 8
VITAMIN C (MG)	20	25	25	30	40
NIACIN (MG) Boys Girls	9 9	13 13	13 13	20 16	23 15
THIAMINE (MG) Boys Girls	0.7 0.7	0.9 0.9	1.0 1.0	1.1 0.9	1.3 0.8
RIBOFLAVIN (MG) Boys Girls	0.8 0.8	1.1 1.1	1.2 1.3	1.5 1.3	1.8 1.3
FOLATE (MCG)	50	70	90	130	200
VITAMIN B$_6$ (MG)	1.0	1.1	1.4	1.7	2.0
VITAMIN B$_{12}$ (MCG)	0.5	0.8	1.0	1.0	1.0
CALCIUM (MG)	500	600	700	1,100	800
IRON (MG) Boys Girls	6 6	8 8	8 8	10 13	10 13
ZINC (MG)	4	5	7	9	12

emphasize fruits, yogurt, or custards instead of pastries and other sweets.

FOODS FOR TODDLERS

After the first year children can eat most of the dishes prepared for the rest of the family. However, because toddlers often have high energy requirements and a small stomach, they may need five or six small meals or snacks a day. Schedule a toddler's snacks so they don't interfere with food intake during meals. An interval of about an hour and a half is usually enough to satisfy hunger without spoiling meals.

Toddlers often go on food jags—for example, eliminating everything that's white or green. Such food rituals are often short-lived, although they can be annoying or worrisome if they get out of hand. Try to respect the child's preferences without giving in to every whim; offer a reasonable alternative. If, for instance, lunch is rejected with a demand for a peanut butter sandwich, resist the temptation to make a substitution but offer to fix the sandwich for a later snack.

BALANCE AND VARIETY

Children need a wide variety of foods. CARBOHYDRATES—breads, cereals, fruits, and vegetables—should make up the major part of the diet. PROTEIN foods can include meat, fish, milk, grains, soy products (such as bean curd), and combinations of grains and legumes. Milk is an important source of calories, minerals, and vitamins. Children 4 to 9 years old should have 2 to 3 milk product servings every day (some of the milk may be in the form of cheese or yogurt). Grilled and baked foods are preferable to fried and fatty ones for children of all ages.

FATS are probably the most misunderstood food group. Although everyone should avoid excess fat, we all need a certain amount for important body functions. Several vitamins (A, D, E, and K) can be absorbed only in

SNACKS AND FAST FOODS

Stock up on healthful snacks that children and teenagers can nibble on throughout the day.

• Breads and crackers with such spreads as peanut butter, low-fat cheese, canned tuna or sardines, and lean cold cuts.

• Rice cakes and whole-grain crackers or breadsticks.

• Fresh and dried fruits.

• Yogurt.

• Sticks of carrot, celery, or other raw vegetables and cherry tomatoes with nutritious dips.

• Plain popcorn.

• Breakfast cereals.

• Water, milk, or fruit juice.

the presence of fat, and fats are necessary for the production of other body chemicals, including the hormones that transform boys and girls into men and women. Excessive fat intake may well lead to obesity and many adult diseases; even so, about 30 percent or less of total calories should come from fat.

Many parents have a battle when it comes to getting children to eat vegetables, but you can win children over by appealing to their taste for bright colors and interesting textures. Who wouldn't choose crisp, raw carrot sticks over soggy, limp cabbage? Innovative cooks can substitute minced vegetables (zucchini, eggplant, mushrooms) for ground meat in spaghetti sauce, or chop chickpeas with grains and other vegetables to make "vegeburgers."

FOODS FOR TEENAGERS

Adolescents need more of everything to keep up with the massive teenage growth spurt: calories and protein for growth and to build muscles; and protein, calcium, phosphorus, and vitamin D for bone formation. For many teenagers the demands of school and social life mean that they eat many meals away from home; suddenly they have the responsibility of choosing perhaps the major part of their diet. Some use food to establish an identity, such as by becoming a VEGETARIAN or going on a diet. Iron-deficiency ANEMIA is fairly common in adolescent girls; the cause is not always clear and may be a problem of absorption rather than the amount of iron in the diet. ANOREXIA and certain other eating disorders are a risk for a small group of adolescents, especially girls.

Obesity (defined as being 20 percent or more above desirable weight) is a problem for both boys and girls, but weight control can be complicated for adolescents. They still need calories for growth, together with the necessary balance of proteins, carbohydrates, and fats. The best approach to controlling weight in obese youngsters is serving smaller portions and encouraging regular, vigorous exercise, which reduces body fat while building lean tissue.

Calcium is important for forming strong, healthy bones during adolescence and preventing osteoporosis later in life. Youths 10 to 16 years old need 3 to 4 milk product servings a day—the equivalent of 2 cups of milk and 1½ ounces (2 slices) of cheese or ¾ cup of yogurt—every day. A rich supply of calcium is found in canned sardines and salmon (where the fish is eaten bones and all), fortified breakfast cereals, and dark green leafy vegetables, such as kale.

Teenagers often prefer snacks loaded with fat, sugar, and salt: potato chips, French fries, hamburgers, hot dogs, pizza, chocolate, and candy bars. These foods are high in sodium and yield a poor balance between calories and nutrition; a steady diet of them is low in vitamins A and C, calcium, and dietary fiber. Encourage teenagers who frequent fast-food restaurants to choose some fresh vegetables and fruits from the salad bar.

Offer your teenager a variety of appealing, healthful snack foods to choose from at home. Teenagers who skip breakfast may start the school day feeling lethargic; slip a breakfast of fruit, cheese, and dried cereal or trail mix into their backpacks to eat on the way to school.

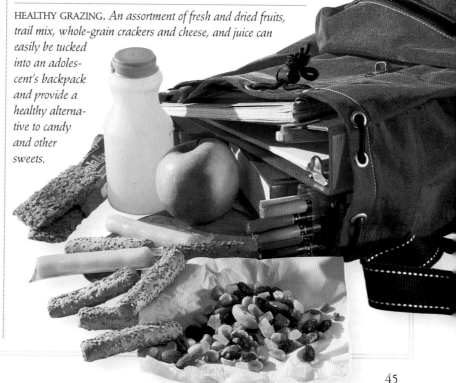

HEALTHY GRAZING. *An assortment of fresh and dried fruits, trail mix, whole-grain crackers and cheese, and juice can easily be tucked into an adolescent's backpack and provide a healthy alternative to candy and other sweets.*

45

CHILIES

BENEFITS
- *An excellent source of vitamins A and C.*
- *May help relieve nasal congestion.*
- *May help prevent blood clots that can lead to a heart attack or stroke.*

DRAWBACKS
- *Require careful handling during preparation to prevent irritation of the skin and eyes.*
- *May irritate hemorrhoids in susceptible people.*

A popular ingredient in Southwestern cooking, chilies, or hot peppers, add spice and interest to many foods; some of the milder varieties are consumed as low-calorie snacks.

The heat in chilies comes from capsaicinoids, substances that have no odor or flavor themselves but impart their bite by acting directly on the mouth's

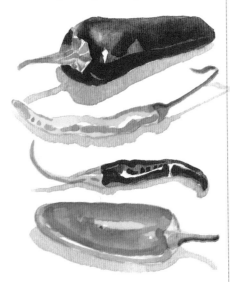

pain receptors. This results in the teary eyes, runny nose ("salsa sniffles"), and sweating experienced by most people who indulge in the hotter varieties. For those with a cold or allergies, eating chilies can provide temporary relief from nasal and sinus congestion. Cap-

A CONSUMERS' GUIDE TO CHILIES

Not all chilies are equally hot; the following is a ranking from the mildest to the hottest.

MILD TO MODERATELY HOT:

- **Anaheim.** These long, slender red or green chilies are among the most popular in the North America.
- **Ancho.** Also called dried poblano, these dark red, heart-shaped peppers are usually dried.
- **Cherry.** These small, round red chilies are often pickled.
- **Poblano.** Green chilies with a small, tapered shape; they are usually roasted, and may be stuffed or added to a variety of dishes.

HOT:

- **Cascabel.** These round red or green chilies are usually dried.

VERY HOT:

- **Cayenne.** These long red chilies are dried and often ground into a hot pepper spice.
- **Habanero.** Shaped like red, yellow, or orange lanterns, these are considered the hottest of cultivated chilies.
- **Jalapeño.** These tapered green or red chilies are sold fresh, canned, or pickled.
- **Serrano.** These small, bullet-shaped green or red chilies are often used in hot salsas.

saicin and other capsaicinoids are concentrated mainly in the white ribs and seeds, which can be removed to produce a milder flavor.

Handle chilies with care. Wear thin gloves and wash all utensils well with soap and water after use. Even a tiny amount of capsaicinoids causes severe irritation if it is transferred to the eyes.

Chilies are more nutritious than sweet peppers, and the red varieties generally have a higher nutritional content than the green ones. They are very good sources of ANTIOXIDANTS, especially vitamins A and C. Just one ounce of chilies contains 70mg of vitamin C, more than 100 percent of the Recommended Nutrient Intake (RNI), as well as about 70 percent of the RNI for vitamin A. Chilies also contain bioflavonoids, plant pigments that some researchers believe may help prevent cancer. In addition, recent research indicates that capsaicin may act as an anticoagulant, perhaps helping to prevent blood clots that can lead to a heart attack or stroke. Incorporated into creams, capsaicinoids alleviate the burning pain of shingles. They may also reduce the mouth pain associated with chemotherapy. Commercially available poultices for relief of lower back also contain capsaicin.

Contrary to popular belief, there is no evidence that chilies can cause ulcers or produce other digestive disturbances. They can, however, cause rectal irritation in some people with hemorrhoids.

CHOCOLATE AND CANDY

BENEFITS
- *Flavorful source of quick energy.*
- *Eating chocolate elevates some people's moods.*

DRAWBACKS
- *Chocolate is high in calories and fat.*
- *Sugary candies can cause tooth decay.*
- *Spoil the appetite for more healthful food choices.*
- *Chocolate may trigger migraine headaches.*
- *Licorice may raise blood pressure in susceptible people.*

Chocolates and candies are nutritionally limited food sources, even though they have been enjoyed by people worldwide for centuries. But despite their nutritional drawbacks, there is no harm in occasionally adding them to an otherwise healthy and balanced diet.

CHOCOLATE

The returning crew of Columbus's fourth voyage in 1502 brought the first cocoa beans from the New World to Europe. The Spanish eventually combined them with vanilla and other flavorings, sugar, and milk to arrive at a concoction that, as one writer noted at the time, people "would die for."

For the first couple of centuries after its introduction in Europe, chocolate was served only as a beverage. A solid form—probably more like marzipan than the chocolate we know—was touted as an instant breakfast in 18th-century France. The stimulant effects of chocolate were thought to make it a particularly useful food for soldiers standing watch during the night.

The chocolate bar, first marketed in about 1910, captured the public imagination when it was issued to the U.S. armed forces as a "fighting food" during World War II.

THE SOURCE OF CHOCOLATE

Chocolate is harvested from the pods and beans of the cocoa tree, an evergreen that originated in the river valleys of South America. Native Central and South Americans valued cocoa so highly that they used cocoa beans as currency. Today about three-fourths of the world's chocolate is grown in West Africa and most of the rest in Brazil.

After cocoa beans are harvested, an initial phase of fermentation and drying is followed by low-temperature roasting to bring out the flavor. Various increasingly complicated manufacturing processes follow, depending on whether the final product is to be solid chocolate or cocoa powder.

In 1828 the Van Houten family of chocolate purveyors in Amsterdam, seeking to make a less-oily drinking chocolate, invented a screw press to remove most of the cocoa butter from the beans. Not only did it make a better drink, but they also found that by mixing the extracted cocoa butter back into ground cocoa beans, they could make a smoother, more unctuous solid paste that would absorb sugar; this eventually led to "eating chocolate."

COMPONENTS

An ounce of solid chocolate contains about 150 calories and 2 or 3 grams of protein. The original bean has significant amounts of vitamin E and the B vitamins. These nutrients, however, are so diluted as to be negligible in modern processed chocolate. Sweet or semi-sweet chocolate contains between 40 and 53 percent fat, or cocoa butter. Both chocolate and cocoa powder supply chromium, iron, magnesium, phosphorus, and potassium, but fat and calories make chocolate an inappropriate source of these minerals except when used in emergency rations.

A chemical composition that prevents it from quickly turning rancid made cocoa butter valuable as a long-lasting food and cosmetic oil.

Chocolate is a solid at room temperature, but since its melting point is just below the human body temperature, it begins to melt and release its flavor components as soon as it is placed in the mouth.

White chocolate, a mixture of cocoa butter, milk solids, and sugar, contains no cocoa solids. Unlike milk chocolate, white chocolate does not keep well, because it lacks the compounds that prevent milk solids from becoming rancid over time.

THE FEEL-GOOD FACTOR

Chocolate contains two related alkaloid stimulants, theobromine and caffeine, in a ratio of about 10 to 1. Theobromine, unlike caffeine, does not stimulate the central nervous system; its effects are mainly diuretic. Commercial chocolate products contain no more than about 0.1 percent caffeine and are much less stimulating, volume for volume, than a cup of decaffeinated coffee. Unsweetened baking chocolate for home use is a more concentrated source of caffeine. Chocolate is also rich in phenylethylamine (PEA), a naturally occurring compound that has effects similar to amphetamine. This compound can also trigger migraine headaches in susceptible people.

Some people (more often women) have a tendency to binge on chocolate after emotional upsets. No scientific basis for this behavior has been proved. However, psychiatrists have theorized that "chocoholics" may be people who have a faulty mechanism for regulating their body levels of phenylethylamine; others attribute chocolate cravings to hormonal changes, such as those that occur during puberty or a woman's premenstrual phase.

After centuries of investigation, chocolate's once-vaunted aphrodisiac qualities can be discounted. But in its

MELTS IN THE MOUTH. *The finest chocolate gets its unique and appealing texture from pure cocoa butter. Its distinct flavor comes from a high proportion of cocoa solids.*

myriad modern forms, chocolate is an endless temptation and, for those who can withstand the caloric assault, a culinary source of pleasure.

CANDY

Our preference for sweet tastes is evident in the womb and is considered to be part of human evolution. For instance, edible berries and fruits tend to be sweet as opposed to the bitter taste of many poisonous plants.

Commercial candy production is believed to have begun when marzipan (a paste made of almonds and sugar) was brought to Italy and Spain through trade with the Arabs and Moors during the Middle Ages. In fact, the word *candy* is derived from the Arabic pronunciation of *khandakah,* the Sanskrit word for sugar.

European candies were first compounded by druggists who preserved herbs in sugar. Candies were rare treats, however, until the widespread cultivation of sugar cane and the development of large-scale refining processes in the 17th and 18th centuries. Modern candies are mostly variations on three basic forms: taffy, from the Creole French word for a mixture of sugar and molasses; nougat, from the Latin word for nutcake; and fondant, from the French for melting (which can be recognized in the texture of fudges and soft-centered chocolates and bars).

NUTRITIONAL DRAWBACKS

All candies are packed with simple sugars—sucrose, corn syrup, fructose—which supply about 375 calories in a 3½-ounce serving and provide quick energy because they are rapidly converted to glucose, or blood sugar. The calorie content of candies varies greatly, however, depending on their other ingredients, such as nuts, fruits, and fat. Although you should count candy calories in your overall daily consumption, don't expect to obtain any useful nutrition from candy.

Practically all hard candies are made with artificial flavors and colorings. In addition, the least expensive candies sold as chocolate often prove to be made of artificial chocolate and vanilla flavoring, with added vegetable fat. It pays to read labels, even with candies, to make sure you know what you're eating.

ADDITIVES AND SENSITIVITIES

There is no scientific evidence that the rigorously tested food dyes allowed in candy by Health Canada cause allergies or adverse reactions in adults or children. These additives are included in minute amounts, and the quantity in an individual serving is not significant. Some people may be hypersensitive to the ingredients in a particular candy, but since candy is not an essential part of the diet, it's easy enough to avoid the offending sweet. Many studies now show that sugar does not cause hyperactivity, but some food dyes in candies

may exacerbate existing hyperactivity.

Natural licorice is known to raise blood pressure in certain people. The effect takes place mainly through the mechanism of salt retention. If you know you're hypertensive, you may be better off avoiding licorice.

SWEETS AND TOOTH DECAY

Sweets and sugary foods form an acid bath that is corrosive to tooth enamel and create an environment where destructive, caries-causing bacteria flourish. The effect is less harmful if you brush your teeth regularly to remove dental plaque. Candies that linger in the mouth are more damaging than those that are quickly swallowed. Chocolate is less likely to cause tooth decay than hard candies. Nevertheless, the sugar in chocolate can do damage.

Sugarless chewing gum is preferable to the sugary kind for adults. (The wisdom of exposing children to artificial sweeteners is questionable.) Gums sweetened with xylitol, a sugar alcohol, have been promoted as "tooth friendly" because xylitol favorably changes the composition and stickiness of dental plaque. When you can't brush after a meal, chewing sugarless gum may help to stimulate the saliva flow and flush food particles out of the mouth. But although gum may be free of caries-inducing sugar, such sweeteners as xylitol and other sugar alcohols typically contain just as many calories as sugar.

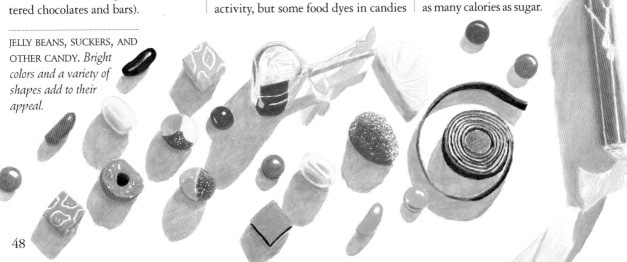

JELLY BEANS, SUCKERS, AND OTHER CANDY. *Bright colors and a variety of shapes add to their appeal.*

CHOLESTEROL: SORTING THE FACTS FROM THE MYTHS

By now, most people know that high levels of blood cholesterol increase the risk of a heart attack. Still, confusion abounds over the role of diet in affecting cholesterol.

Although often portrayed as a dietary pariah, cholesterol is essential to life. The body needs it to make sex hormones, bile, vitamin D, cell membranes, and nerve sheaths. These and other functions fall to serum cholesterol, a waxy, fatlike compound that circulates in the bloodstream. The liver manufactures about a gram each day, which is all the body requires.

Dietary cholesterol is found only in animal products. The body does not need this cholesterol, but anyone other than a strict VEGETARIAN who excludes all animal products will consume varying amounts of it. Many factors—exercise, genetics, gender, and other components of the diet—influence how the human body processes dietary cholesterol; some people can consume large amounts but have normal blood levels, while others eat very little but have high blood cholesterol.

GOOD VS. BAD CHOLESTEROL

To travel through the bloodstream, cholesterol molecules attach themselves to lipid-carrying proteins, or lipoproteins. Two types of lipoproteins are the major transporters of cholesterol: low-density lipoproteins (LDLs) carry two-thirds of it; most of the remainder is attached to high-density lipoproteins (HDLs). LDLs tend to deposit cholesterol in the artery walls, leading to atherosclerosis and an increased risk of heart disease. In contrast, HDLs collect cholesterol from the artery walls and other tissues and take it to the liver to be metabolized and eliminated from the body. This is why LDLs are often called the "bad" cholesterol and HDLs the "good." A third type, very-low-density lipoproteins, VLDLs, carry a small amount of cholesterol and triglycerides.

A blood cholesterol test measures the amount of cholesterol in the blood. This can be expressed in terms of milligrams (mg) of cholesterol per deciliter or millimoles (mmol) of cholesterol per liter. The multiplication factor 0.026 converts the milligram system to the millimole system. A value below 200mg/dl (5.2 mmol/l) is considered desirable. If the total is more than 200mg, LDL and HDL levels should be measured individually. LDL levels should be below 130mg/dl; 130 to 159 is classified as borderline high, over 160 is considered high risk for coronary artery disease and a heart attack. HDL levels should be at least 45mg/dl, and the higher the better. In assessing cardiovascular risk, doctors calculate the LDL/HDL ratio by dividing the total cholesterol by the HDL figure. A desirable ratio is less than 4.5. For example, if your total cholesterol is 220 and your HDL level is 55, then your ratio is 4.0, putting you in a low-risk category.

HOW DIET CAN HELP

Experts agree that dietary modification is appropriate if the total cholesterol count is greater than 200mg/dl (5.2 mmol/l) or if the LDL level exceeds 130mg/dl (3.4 mmol/l). Reducing intake of saturated FATS has the greatest effect on lowering blood cholesterol levels. A diet that limits fat intake to 20 percent or less of total calories and restricts saturated fats to 7 percent or less can lower total blood cholesterol an average of 14 percent. Most people can significantly lower intake of saturated fats by cutting down on or eliminating fatty meats, whole milk and other dairy products, and baked goods made with tropical (coconut, palm, and palm kernel) oils.

Stricter diets yield even better results. For example, the vegetarian low-fat (less than 10 percent of calories) program developed by Dr. Dean Ornish can lower LDL cholesterol by up to 70mg/dl. The Ornish program also calls for daily exercise and meditation.

It isn't just what you don't eat that matters; consuming foods that have a cholesterol-lowering effect also helps. Oat bran and dried beans and peas are high in a soluble fiber, which lowers cholesterol. The pectin in apples and other fruits also lowers cholesterol, as does, apparently, the soy protein found in tofu, tempeh, and soy milk.

Two or three servings a week of salmon, sardines, shrimp, lobster, and other cold-water fish or seafood are linked with a reduced risk of heart attacks and strokes. Initially, it was thought that the omega-3 fatty acids in seafood reduced cardiovascular risk by lowering blood cholesterol levels; however, recent studies suggest that their benefit comes from interfering with blood clotting and from possible changes in the way the liver metabolizes other lipids.

At one time, increasing the intake of polyunsaturated fats—corn, cottonseed, safflower, soy, and sunflower oils—was advocated to lower cholesterol, but more recent studies have found that these oils reduce the levels of the protective HDLs while having little effect on the harmful LDLs. In contrast, monounsaturated fats found in canola and olive oils have the opposite effect, cutting LDLs without altering HDL levels.

The role of dietary cholesterol is still unclear; recent studies indicate it is not as potent in raising blood cholesterol as saturated fats are (see Eating to Keep Cholesterol in Check, right). Still, some experts recommend limiting dietary cholesterol intake to 300mg a day—the amount in one and one-half egg yolks, 4 ounces of beef liver, or a combination of 2 cups of whole milk (60mg), a 6-ounce steak (180mg), and 1 cup of ice cream (60mg).

OTHER APPROACHES

Increased exercise, weight loss, and stress reduction can all lower cholesterol or improve the LDL/HDL ratio. Women are protected from developing coronary artery disease during their reproductive years by estrogen, and new research indicates that postmenopausal hormone replacement extends this protection into old age.

Moderate ALCOHOL intake lowers the risk of heart attack. This may be due to alcohol's ability to raise HDL, its tendency to reduce the stickiness of platelets, or the presence of antioxidants, such as resveratrol, in red wine.

If dietary and other lifestyle changes fail to reduce blood cholesterol, drugs may be prescribed.

EATING TO KEEP CHOLESTEROL IN CHECK

There's no doubt that what you eat influences the levels of cholesterol and other lipids in your blood. Numerous studies document that diets high in animal products and other saturated fats tend to elevate cholesterol levels, in contrast to the low levels found in people whose diets consist largely of starches, fruits, and vegetables. Individuals with a family history of heart disease should be diligent in structuring a diet that limits the cholesterol-raising foods and emphasizes the cholesterol-lowering foods indicated below.

FOODS THAT MAY RAISE CHOLESTEROL

Hard margarine and vegetable shortening, which are high in saturated fats and trans fatty acids.

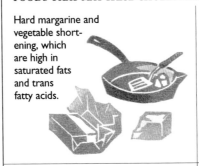

Fatty meat and meat products, such as marbled beef, pork and lamb chops, hamburgers, bacon, frankfurters, salamis, and other cold cuts.

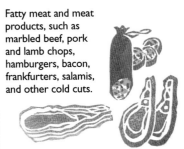

Cookies, cakes, pastries, and chocolates, especially those made with saturated tropical oils.

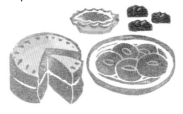

Dairy products, such as cheese, cream, and butter, which are high in saturated fats.

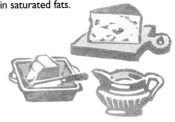

FOODS THAT MAY LOWER CHOLESTEROL

Whole-wheat, pumpernickel, rye, and multigrain bread and rolls.

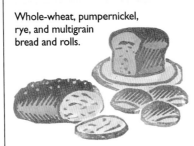

Fruits, such as oranges, apples, pears, bananas, and such dried fruits as apricots, figs, and prunes.

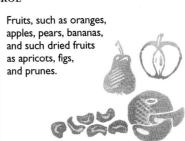

Oatmeal and breakfast cereals that contain oat or rice bran, as well as tofu and other soy products.

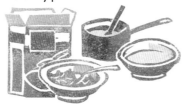

Vegetables, such as sweet corn, onions, garlic, lima beans, kidney beans, and other legumes.

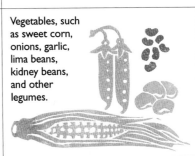

EYE DISORDERS

CONSUME PLENTY OF

- *Carrots, sweet potatoes, and dark green vegetables for beta carotene.*
- *Citrus fruits, melons, tomatoes, and dark green vegetables for vitamin C.*
- *Whole grains, seeds, nuts, green vegetables, avocados, potatoes, bananas, fish, poultry, and lean meat for B vitamins.*
- *Vegetable oils, wheat germ, liver, fish, fresh green leafy vegetables, legumes, and dried fruits for vitamin E.*
- *Whole-grain cereals, seafood, lean meat, poultry, and eggs for selenium and zinc.*

CUT DOWN ON

- *Saturated fats.*

The role of ANTIOXIDANT nutrients and bioflavonoids in vision loss and other degenerative problems associated with aging is becoming increasingly clear. With advancing age, the production of free radicals, unstable molecules that form when the body uses oxygen, increases. These molecules cause eye damage like that which results from exposure to radiation, and contribute to such degenerative disorders as cataracts and macular degeneration.

AGE-RELATED DISORDERS

Cataracts develop when the lens—the transparent membrane that allows light to enter the eye—yellows, hindering the passage of light rays through it. Vision becomes hazy, cloudy, or blurry; if untreated, the lens may become completely opaque, resulting in blindness.

Although aging is the most common cause of cataracts, they can occur at any time of life, even in infancy. Smoking and diabetes can hasten their development. But a diet that provides ample antioxidants—in particular, vitamins C and E and the mineral selenium—appears to slow their progression.

Another eye disease that comes with aging, macular degeneration, is one of the most common causes of legal blindness among older North Americans. It entails a gradual, painless deterioration of the macula, tissue in the central portion of the retina. The first symptom is usually blurring of central vision; eventually, the person may have only limited side vision. The cause of macular degeneration is unknown, but recent research suggests that a diet high in antioxidant nutrients may help prevent or slow the disorder.

Some studies also suggest that riboflavin and vitamin B_6 may help protect the eyes from age-related macular degeneration. Research also shows that a diet high in saturated fats increases the risk of age-related macular degeneration. Scientists theorize that saturated fats may clog the arteries in the retina in the same way that they contribute to atherosclerosis in larger blood vessels, such as the coronary arteries.

DIABETIC RETINOPATHY

Certain similarities between macular degeneration and diabetic retinopathy—the infiltration of the retina with tiny ruptured blood vessels—suggest that antioxidant nutrients may also be beneficial in this common complication of diabetes. Diet is critical in maintaining tight control of blood glucose levels, which also reduces the risk of diabetic retinopathy. A diet high in starches, fruits, and vegetables, with moderate amounts of protein and minimal fat, not only keeps diabetes in check but may also help prevent eye damage and the other serious complications of the disease.

NIGHT BLINDNESS

The eyes need vitamin A and its precursor, beta carotene, as well as bioflavonoids, to make the pigments that absorb light within the eye. A deficiency in vitamin A or a failure to utilize it properly impairs the eye's ability to adapt to darkness and leads to night blindness. This does not entail a total loss of night vision, but rather difficulty seeing well in dim lighting.

Vitamin A deficiency is uncommon in Western industrialized countries, but it remains a major problem in many underdeveloped areas of the world. Organ meats, fortified margarine, butter, and other dairy products are good sources of vitamin A. Dark yellow or orange foods, such as carrots, sweet potatoes, and apricots, as well as dark green leafy vegetables, are the richest sources of beta carotene, which the body converts to vitamin A.

Failing night vision should not be self-treated with vitamin A or beta carotene supplements; the problem may stem from a digestive or malabsorption disorder that prevents the body from using the vitamin. Treatment of the underlying cause usually cures the night blindness. An exception is night blindness caused by retinitis pigmentosa, a genetic disease. However, recent research suggests that vitamin A may, in fact, slow the progressive vision loss of this incurable disease.

CONJUNCTIVITIS

Commonly called pink eye, conjunctivitis is an irritation or infection of the membrane that lines the front of the eyeball and eyelid. Typical symptoms include redness, itchiness, a burning sensation, a thin watery discharge, and a yellow crust that forms during sleep.

Viruses are responsible for most conjunctivitis, but in recurring cases an ALLERGIC REACTION may be the cause. Some people, for example, suffer conjunctivitis as part of hay fever; others react to certain foods. If you suspect a food is causing the conjunctivitis, try eliminating that food from your diet for a few weeks. If the eye irritation disappears only to return when you reintroduce the food into your diet, you have probably identified the offending culprit, which you can then avoid.

FAD DIETS

Each year, yet another miracle diet comes on the scene.
Despite all the hype and claims, none ever lives up to its
promises of painless weight loss and renewed health.

Canadians spend more than $300 million each year on commercial weight-loss programs, and experts agree that this is not only a waste of money but also a threat to health. Most fad diets promise fast weight loss, but some address other concerns: Some play on common misconceptions (the body needs to be detoxified periodically) or groundless fears (our foods are filled with harmful additives or fail to provide essential nutrients). Other diets are outgrowths of religious or philosophical tenets—for example, macrobiotic or Ayurvedic regimens.

In general, purveyors of fad diets take advantage of a person's insecurity about what constitutes good nutrition. Some have medical degrees, but many are naturopaths (self-styled nutritionists) who appear sincere but whose real goal is to sell special dietary products. You should be wary of any regimen that rejects the principles outlined in BASIC FOOD GROUPS or makes unrealistic promises. Although a nutritious, balanced diet is necessary to maintain health, no diet or supplement will cure cancer or restore lost youth. Be cautious, too, of regimens driven by an obvious profit motive; for example, any that require membership fees, costly books or supplements, special food, or exercise equipment. These are often sold through television infomercials or by telephone solicitors.

Before undertaking any major dietary change, it's a good idea to check with a doctor, registered dietitian, or qualified nutritionist. These professionals can quickly ascertain whether a diet is nutritionally sound.

CRASH WEIGHT LOSS

At any given time, more than 3 million Canadians are on some kind of weight-loss diet, and a similar number either plan to diet or think they should. All too often these dieters turn to some sort of crash plan that promises fast results. In recent years there have been the Scarsdale, Fit for Life, Bloomingdale's, Hamptons, Aspen, Mediterranean, Atkins, Stillman, Air Force, grapefruit, rice, drinking man's, high-fat, pasta, high-fiber, high-protein, water, chocolate-lover's, cabbage soup, and macrobiotic diets—to name a few.

All these diets promise relatively painless weight loss; indeed, most people will lose weight if they follow any one for more than a few weeks. Although the focus varies from one diet to another, they all restrict the total intake of calories, including diets that proclaim you can eat all you want. In most of these diets, the food choices tend to be limited and so boring that there's little temptation to overeat. The fruits and rice diet, for example, allows for large amounts of most fresh fruits and moderate portions of rice. After a few days of this monotonous fare, most people are so sick of fruits and rice that they end up eating even less than the diet's allotted portions.

This restricted approach to dieting and weight control not only carries a risk of nutritional deficiencies but is doomed to failure, because it does not instill a permanent change in eating habits. As soon as former eating habits are resumed, the unwanted weight is rapidly regained.

Losing weight often becomes more difficult with each successive attempt; this is commonly referred to as the yo-yo effect. If a person seriously wants to lose weight and keep it off, the only truly successful way is to adopt sensible, permanent exercise and diet habits that balance food intake with expended energy.

COMMON DIET MYTHS

Many alternative practitioners recommend periodic detoxification diets; they believe that these diets cleanse the digestive system and rid the body of waste products. A typical detoxification regimen calls for a few days of fasting, during which the person consumes only distilled water, fruit juice, raw fruit, and perhaps spirula (a type of algae), bran, various supplements, and herbs or herbal teas. In many regimens, enemas are advocated to further cleanse the colon, as well as saunas or sweat baths to rid the body of "toxins" through the skin. Some practitioners also recommend chelation, which entails administering a drug that binds with minerals to remove them from the body.

There is no scientific evidence that the body needs detoxification—it has its own highly efficient waste-removal systems. Indeed, detoxification regimens not only upset the body's natural waste removal, they can also be harmful. Enemas disrupt normal colon function and can upset the body's natural chemical balance. Fasting, especially during an illness, deprives the body of the energy and nutrients it needs to heal itself. Chelation therapy is justified in cases of lead, mercury, or other metal poisoning, but not in the treatment of arthritis, atherosclerosis, and other diseases.

DIET AND PHILOSOPHY

Most religion-based dietary regimens are generally healthy; in fact, studies show that people who follow the vegetarian regimens of Seventh-Day Adventists or Buddhists often live longer and enjoy a lower incidence of obesity, heart disease, cancer, and other serious diseases than do those who consume a typical Western diet.

This doesn't apply to some restrictive diets, such as the most extreme levels of the macrobiotic regimen. In the 1900s the macrobiotic diet was developed by the American-Japanese writer George Ohsawa, who credited the diet with curing his tuberculosis. His dietary system classified all foods according to the Chinese system of opposing forces, as yin or yang, instead of using protein, carbohydrate, and fat designations. The philosophy is to balance foods according to their yin and yang qualities. Foods should also be seasonal and locally grown. Geography and methods of preparation, too, are classified as yin and yang; for example, a person living in a warm (yang) area should emphasize yin foods, and vice versa. Yin foods should predominate during the warm summer months, yang foods during the winter months.

There are seven increasingly restricted levels of macrobiotics. Brown rice and herbal teas are basic items in all levels. Grains, vegetables, and fruits make up the bulk of the diet; fish and some meat are permitted on the lower levels, dairy products and all processed foods are avoided on every level.

The liberal, lower-level macrobiotic diets are low-fat, mostly vegetarian regimens that meet all or most of our nutritional needs. In contrast, the extreme upper-level macrobiotic diets are deficient in many nutrients, such as vitamin B_{12}, iron, and calcium.

Warning: Long-term use of the extreme upper-level diets can result in anemia and other deficiency diseases. Some alternative practitioners recommend a limited macrobiotic regimen for AIDS and cancer patients—a practice that may prove dangerous. People with these life-threatening diseases generally need more, not less, nutrition. A strict macrobiotic diet should also be avoided by a pregnant or breast-feeding woman, children, or anyone needing extra calories.

MACROBIOTIC STAPLES

There are seven levels of macrobiotic diet. The less extreme levels are mainly vegetarian (although they may allow fish and some meat), consisting of large amounts of unrefined cereals and small amounts of seasonal and locally produced fruits and vegetables. The most extreme level, now rarely followed, consists of brown rice only. Several deaths from malnutrition have been attributed to this regimen. A suitable macrobiotic diet can include the following foods:

Whole-grain cereals. Brown rice, oats, barley, wheat, buckwheat, corn, rye, millet, and products made from these, such as whole-wheat flour, bread, and pasta; couscous; oatmeal.

Fruits. A mixture of fresh seasonal fruits, which should include some citrus fruits. To ensure freshness, buy frequently and, where possible, choose local produce.

Vegetables and seaweed. A wide variety of fresh vegetables is recommended. Seaweed is used to enhance the flavor and nutritional value of many dishes.

Legumes. Lentils, chickpeas, beans, peas, and soy products, such as tofu (bean curd).

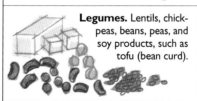

Soups. Often made with beans, lentils, and special Asian seasonings, such as miso (made from fermented soya beans), shoyu (a dark soy sauce), and dried seaweed.

Seeds, nuts, flavorings, and fish. Sesame, sunflower, and pumpkin seeds, peanuts, almonds, hazelnuts, walnuts, and dried chestnuts. In moderation, sea salt, ginger, mustard, tahini, cider vinegar, garlic, lemon juice, and apple juice can all be used to enhance the flavor of a dish. For nonvegetarians, three small portions of fresh seafood can be included every week. The yang qualities of fish and shellfish should be balanced by helpings of green leafy vegetables, grains, or legumes at the same meal.

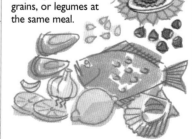

FATS: AN ABUNDANCE OF FACTS AND FALLACIES

Each year brings a new tide of conflicting information about fats. Some claims are false, others are based on incomplete data, yet still others raise important health concerns.

In all the debate about dietary fats, there are three facts beyond dispute: one, in small amounts, fats are essential to maintain health; two, the typical North American diet is much too high in fats of all kinds; and three, the fat debate is a gold mine for commercial exploitation of the popular pursuit of low-fat and fat-free alternatives to traditional foods.

BENEFITS
- *Supply the fatty acids the body needs for many chemical activities, including growth, metabolism, and the manufacture of sex hormones and cell membranes.*
- *Transport the fat-soluble vitamins A, D, E, and K in the body.*
- *Add flavor, aroma, and smooth, pleasing texture to foods, making eating more enjoyable.*
- *Satisfy feelings of hunger.*
- *An important source of energy for basal metabolism.*

DRAWBACKS
- *A high-fat diet easily leads to weight gain.*
- *Saturated fat is linked to elevated blood cholesterol levels and an increased risk of heart disease, stroke, and circulatory disorders.*
- *A high fat intake may increase the risk of developing certain cancers, particularly of the colon, prostate, breast, and ovaries.*

Lipids is the term applied interchangeably to fats, oils, waxes, sterols, esters, and similar substances that usually cannot be dissolved in water but will dissolve in an organic solvent. Dietary fats and oils are members of the same chemical family, the triglycerides. They differ in their melting points: at room temperature, fats are solid, whereas oils are liquid. In other respects they can be considered as a single class of compounds, and for simplicity can be referred to as fats.

Natural fats, whether they are derived from animal or plant sources, are composed of three fatty acid molecules (a triglyceride) bound by one glycerol (a type of alcohol) molecule. The nature of a fat depends on which specific combination of fatty acids is drawn from a basic pool of about 25.

All fats contain the same number of calories by weight; that is, about 250 calories per ounce, or 9 calories per gram. Volume for volume, however, the calorie count can differ substantially. For example, a cup of oil weighs more—and therefore has more calories—than a cup of whipped margarine, into which air has been added to increase its volume. In addition, if the whipped margarine is one of the low-calorie versions, a considerable percentage of its weight will come from added water.

A diet rich in high-fat foods results in more weight gain than a diet made up mainly of carbohydrates with some protein. Not only are fats a more concentrated source of calories than the other food groups, but recent studies indicate that the body is also more efficient in storing fats than carbohydrates and protein.

HOW WE USE FATS

It is important to distinguish the fat consumed in foods—dietary fat—from body fats circulating in the blood or stored as adipose tissue, which is made up of cells specially adapted for that purpose. Even if the diet contains no fat whatsoever, the body will convert any excess protein and carbohydrate to fat and store them as such. When our weight remains steady, it's because we are making fat and using it up at equal rates. If our food intake exceeds our need for energy, then no matter what the composition of the diet, we synthesize more fat than we use and gain weight.

The average woman's body is about 20 to 25 percent fat by weight; the average man's is 15 percent. The greater proportion of fat in women is an evolutionary adaptation to meet the demand for extra calories needed to bear and nourish children.

Most body cells have a limited capacity for fat storage. The fat cells (adipocytes) are exceptions; they expand as more fat accumulates. An obese person's fat cells may be 50 to 100 times larger than those of a thin person. In addition, overweight infants

THE FAMILY TREE OF FATS

Fats and oils contain many different fatty acids that affect the body in varying ways. Most simply, they are classified as saturated or unsaturated based on their molecular structure.

Unsaturates are further subdivided into monounsaturates and polyunsaturates. Trans fatty acids are created in food processing and also occur naturally in beef, lamb, and dairy products.

THE FATS IN EVERYDAY FOODS

Saturated fatty acids. Butter, hard cheese, and palm and coconut oils. Fatty meat products also have a high percentage of saturated fats.

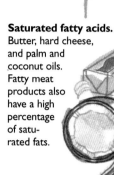

Monounsaturated fatty acids. The principal sources are olive oil, canola oil, and such foods as avocados, nuts, and seeds. Olive oil, canola oil, and some nuts also contain important polyunsaturates.

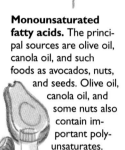

Polyunsaturated fatty acids. Foods high in polyunsaturated fats include corn and most other vegetable oils, fish oils, and oily fish. These also have two types of essential fatty acids.

Trans fatty acids. Hydrogenated oils, such as margarine; fats that are industrially hardened to avoid rancidity; and processed foods, such as pies, cakes, and potato and other chips, are the major sources of trans fatty acids.

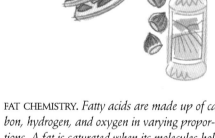

Omega-6 (linoleic acid and its derivatives). Good sources include corn, safflower, soybean, and sunflower oils.

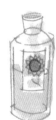

Omega-3 (linolenic acid and its derivatives). Good sources include rapeseed and evening primrose oils, flaxseed, walnuts, and oily fish, such as sardines, mackerel, and salmon.

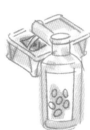

FAT CHEMISTRY. *Fatty acids are made up of carbon, hydrogen, and oxygen in varying proportions. A fat is saturated when its molecules hold the maximum amount of hydrogen. Monounsaturates have a little less, while polyunsaturates have the least. Trans fatty acids can be created by the hydrogenation process.*

and children accumulate more fat cells than their thin counterparts. Once in place, fat cells will never go away, although they will shrink if fat is drawn off to be used for energy production. One theory has it that shrunken fat cells emit a chemical plea for replenishment, which could explain why many people spend their lives on a roller coaster of weight loss and gain.

WHY WE NEED FATS

Fats add flavor and a smooth, pleasing texture to foods. Because they take longer to digest, fats continue to let us feel full even after the proteins and carbohydrates have been emptied from the stomach. Fats also stimulate the intestine to release cholecystokinin, a hormone that suppresses the appetite and signals us to stop eating.

Stored body fats provide a fuel reserve for future needs—one pound of body fat provides enough energy to last 1½ to 2 days. The chemical structure of fats allows them to store about twice as much energy in a given weight as carbohydrates do. This means that if a 120-pound woman's fat supply were converted into its energy equivalent in carbohydrates, her weight would balloon to 150 pounds.

The layer of fat just beneath the skin (about half of the total stored amount) provides insulation against changes in temperature. While very thin people may be oversensitive to cold, those carrying extra fat often suffer more in hot weather. This subcutaneous fat is also instrumental in the manufacture of vitamin D when the skin is exposed to the sun.

Deposits of fat that surround the vital organs hold them in place and help cushion them against injury. These protective deposits are among the last to be depleted if the body's energy stores run low.

REDUCING YOUR FAT INTAKE

• Limit meat to 3 or 4 ounces per serving. Buy lean cuts that contain no more than 9 percent fat (look for products that state fat content on the label). Trim all visible fat before cooking. Buy extra-lean ground beef, or better still, select a lean cut and ask the butcher to grind it for you.

• Remove the skin from poultry before eating it. (In some instances, this can be done before cooking.)

• Don't buy prebasted turkey; it's often injected with coconut oil, butter, or other fats.

• Broil, bake, or roast meat, fish, and poultry. Use a roasting rack to drain off the fat as the meat cooks.

• Cook stews and soups in advance; chill and skim off the congealed fat, and reheat before serving.

• Avoid fried foods. Use a nonstick pan and vegetable oil spray for sautéing.

• Buy low-fat (1 percent) or skim milk, low-fat cheese and cottage cheese, and fat-free yogurt.

• Toss salad with fat-free dressings or make your own with lemon juice or vinegar, mustard, herbs, and spices. If oil is called for, use olive oil.

• Buy a low-fat or even a fat-free substitute for mayonnaise.

• Cook rice in a fat-free broth; flavor it with chopped fresh herbs and scallions instead of butter.

• Mash potatoes with low-fat yogurt or buttermilk; add chives and parsley for extra zip.

• Serve higher-fat foods in smaller portions; compensate with larger servings of low-fat items, such as pasta, vegetables, and fruits.

• Eliminate the use of nondairy creamers and toppings; these products are usually high in saturated fats because they are made with palm oil or coconut oil.

• Serve fat-free frozen yogurt instead of ice cream or consider other fat-free dessert alternatives, such as fresh fruits, and gelatins, and angel food cake.

Fats also supply the fatty acids that are essential for numerous chemical processes, including growth and development in children, the production of sex hormones and prostaglandins (hormonelike chemicals that are responsible for regulating many body processes), the formation and function of cell membranes, and the transport of other molecules into and out of the cells. Interestingly enough, fat does not supply energy for the brain and nervous system, both of which rely on glucose for fuel. Like certain vitamins and amino acids, some fatty acids must be obtained from the diet, because the body cannot synthesize them. As a result, our need for essential fatty acids is met by linoleic acid (found in vegetable oils, especially corn, safflower, and soybean oils), which is then converted in the body into arachidonic acid, an essential fatty acid. Finally, fats are needed for the transport and absorption of the fat-soluble vitamins A, D, E, and K.

DIETARY INTAKE

In developing countries fats make up 10 percent of daily calories. In North America daily fat intake has increased from about 30 percent of the daily diet 100 years ago to 35 to 40 percent today. This is the equivalent of approximately a fifth of a pound of pure fat a day and is more than six to eight times what we actually need. The Heart and Stroke Foundation of Canada recommends that adults restrict their total fat intake to no more than 30 percent of each day's calories. Some authorities believe this should be lowered to 20 percent, but others feel this is an unrealistic goal for most people. For healthy children over the age of 2, The Canadian Paediatric Society recommends a diet that provides no more than 30 percent of energy as fat, and no more than 10 percent of energy as saturated fat, which is needed for growth and proper brain development.

A tablespoon of vegetable oil provides enough linoleic acid and fat to transport all the fat-soluble vitamins we need in a day; any more than this is unnecessary. Reducing dietary fat is difficult, however, as two-thirds of it is hidden in lean meat, cheese, fried foods, sauces, nuts, pastries, and so on. (See Reducing Your Fat Intake, left.)

SATURATION

The types of fats consumed may be more important than total fat intake. For years nutritionists have recommended unsaturated over saturated fats (see The Family Tree of Fats, p.55). In general, saturated fats (but not palm, palm kernel, and coconut oils) are solid at room temperature; most animal fats (beef, butter, and cheeses) are saturated. Monounsaturated fats are liquid at room temperature and solid or semi-solid under refrigeration (margarine and olive and peanut oils). Polyunsaturated fats are liquid (corn and sunflower oils) unless hydrogen is added in the process called hydrogenation, as in the manufacture of margarine.

Highly saturated fats raise blood CHOLESTEROL levels because they interfere with the removal of cholesterol from the blood. Monounsaturated and polyunsaturated fats, by contrast, either lower blood cholesterol or have no effect on it. When polyunsaturated fats are hydrogenated to make them firm, they become like saturated fats in their effects on blood cholesterol.

Cutting down on saturated fats involves choosing vegetable fats over animal fats and favoring monounsaturates over polyunsaturates. Remember that a food labeled as 95 percent fat free may still derive most of its calories from fat. The fat free calculation is based on total weight which includes the weight of water in the food.

REGIONAL DIETS AND HOW THEY IMPACT ON HEALTH

In an attempt to pinpoint a cause of heart disease, diabetes, and certain cancers that are so prevalent in Western societies, researchers are increasingly looking at data from other cultures whose diets are quite different from our own.

The Japanese Diet

It is no coincidence that the Japanese, whose diet contains just over 30 percent fat (mostly polyunsaturated), compared with 35 to 40 per-

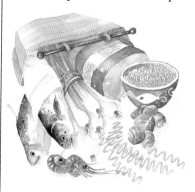

cent in North America—and even more in Britain, Germany, and many other European countries—should enjoy one of the lowest rates of heart disease in the world.

Japanese cuisine emphasizes fish in such forms as sushi, sashimi, and tempura; on average, the Japanese consume 100g (3.5 ounces) of fish a day. The staple food, however, is rice. A basic meal includes steamed rice, soup (such as miso, made with soybean paste), and small side dishes that may contain meat, vegetables (including seaweed), seafoods, fish, eggs, chicken, and noodles, in different sauces and combinations.

As in the West, the Japanese eat three meals a day. Traditionally, breakfast consists of rice and a miso soup made of such ingredients as seaweed, tofu, or leeks, and a side dish, such as grilled fish. A typical lunch might be chicken and vegetables cooked in a soup stock blended with eggs and served on rice. Dinner, the most important meal of the day, might include a small portion of grilled fish as well as a meat dish, such as stewed beef and bean sprouts, served with boiled greens, miso soup, and rice.

The Mediterranean Diet

Although people living in France, Greece, Spain, and Italy eat slightly more fat than North Americans, most of it is unsaturated. Amazingly, their risk of fatal heart disease is less than half that of North Americans.

The staple foods of the Mediterranean countries are rice, bread, potatoes, pasta, and cereals, such as couscous, accompanied by plenty of vegetables. Olive oil is widely used in cooking; other sources of fat include nuts, seeds, and oily fish, such as sardines. It should be noted that butter consumption in Spain, Portugal, Italy, and Greece (but not in France) is relatively low.

The Mediterranean breakfast is light, often made up of rolls, coffee, and fruit juice or fruit. Lunch may

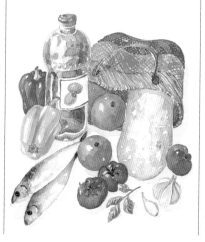

include a protein dish of meat, fish, or poultry, bread or pasta, and sometimes a vegetable. Dinner is often an extended meal of several courses, accompanied by wine. At both lunch and dinner, salad is served, often as a separate course.

People living in southern Europe eat more legumes, nuts, and vegetables than North Americans; on average the Mediterranean diet includes five or more servings of fruits and vegetables a day.

The Western Diet

The typical diet in Canada and other industrialized countries is high in saturated fats from animal sources.

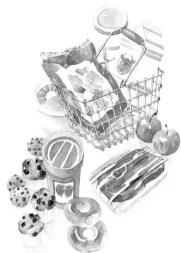

North Americans tend to eat two or more portions of meat, fish, or poultry a day and drink a pint or more of milk or its equivalent in cheese, yogurt, or other milk products. Other popular sources of fat include butter or margarine, mayonnaise, and snack foods, especially potato chips, French fries, ice cream, and baked goods. People are now eating more vegetables, fruits, and starchy foods, but still less than the recommended amounts.

HOSPITAL DIETS: MEALS FOR CONVALESCENTS

*Many illnesses and medical treatments can cause
nutrition and feeding problems. Meanwhile, good nutrition
is essential for getting better and staying healthy.*

Balanced nutrition is especially important during periods of illness and convalescence. Many illnesses can result in nutrient deficiency, increasing the need for nourishment at a time when it is hard for patients to consume adequate amounts of food. A balanced diet can enhance the sense of well-being as well as prospects for recovery in people with cancer, those undergoing surgery, victims of severe burns, alcoholics, and patients with other conditions.

Another problem is that periods of prolonged bed rest weaken the muscles and bones, and contribute to the risk of blood clots in the deep veins. Exercise programs should be designed (even for bedridden patients) to maintain muscle tone, bone strength, and a brisk flow of circulation.

Attitudes to convalescence have undergone radical revision. Now, even after extensive surgery or an acute crisis, a prolonged period of enforced rest is rarely recommended. Rather, doctors encourage patients to resume normal activities, with realistic lifestyle changes that can be maintained for a lifetime of renewed good health.

EATING TO GET WELL

Diets for hospitalized patients, as well as for those being cared for at home, should complement medical and surgical treatment. For most patients, no special measures are necessary; they can recover on the hospital or family diet with only minor changes, where appropriate, in a few nutrients (such as sodium) or calorie content.

Good nutrition is especially important for people who are likely to remain in the hospital for extended periods. Studies have shown that patients can incur nutritional problems in the course of hospitalization, regardless of their status on admission. Malnutrition can develop during prolonged (5 to 7 days) administration of intravenous fluids without nutrient supplementation. Also, patients may suffer a loss of nutrients as a result of medical procedures, such as kidney dialysis, or specific symptoms, such as diarrhea. Extra energy is needed for healing and for fighting infection or fever. Finally, medications and treatments (typically, steroids, chemotherapy, and radiation) can interfere with the intake or metabolism of nutrients.

When a patient has special needs, hospital dietitians will devise an eating plan to include one or more of the following goals: to correct a nutritional deficiency; to compensate for the body's inability to handle certain nutrients; or to spare a specific organ by changing the form of nutrients or the timing of meals. Hospital diets can be further adjusted for patients with religious or personal preferences. Make your needs known at the time of hospital admission; include allergies and food intolerances and any vitamins or nonprescription drugs you may be taking. If the meals served are unsatisfactory, ask if alternative choices are available or if food may be brought in from outside the hospital.

When the nutrition plan represents a permanent change of eating habits or one that should be maintained for an extended period, the hospital should provide printed guidelines for preparing meals at home. Before leaving the hospital, make an appointment with a dietitian. In this way, you can find out if substitutions are allowed and how far you can bend the rules in order to increase variety in the diet.

As a caregiver, you can ask for the nutritionist's advice, too; you may have difficulty in weaning a patient from hospital liquids to solid foods, or you may need help in adjusting to a new form of feeding for special needs.

Planning for those continuing treatment should take medicine-food interactions into consideration. Certain drugs can influence the absorption of nutrients, and a variety of nutrients affect the absorption of medications or alter the metabolism of drugs in the liver.

NUTRITION ALTERNATIVES

When patients cannot eat enough to meet their needs, doctors may order supplemental nutrition or feeding by an alternative route. At the basic level, a doctor may suggest larger portions or the use of nutrient-enriched drinks. Easy to eat and digest, these relatively high-calorie liquids may be fortified with protein, vitamins, and minerals. For those who haven't the time or resources to prepare supplemental foods at home, commercial formulas are available. It's important to keep supplements in their proper place, however; most will provide only selected nutrients and are not meant to take the place of solid food or a balanced diet. When a patient is restricted to liquid feeding alone, the doctor will specify a formula to cover complete nutritional requirements.

For patients who can absorb and digest food but cannot take enough nourishment by mouth, tube feeding—called enteral feeding—may be necessary. Most people need enteral feeding for only a limited time, but some must continue it indefinitely. A tube is usually threaded through the nose and into the digestive tract; this is called a nasogastric tube. In some cases, the tube may be inserted directly into the stomach (gastrostomy) or into the small intestine.

When enteral feeding is inadequate or impossible, parenteral (meaning outside the digestive tract) nutrition is given through a catheter directly into the bloodstream. Parenteral nutrition is sometimes used to spare the digestive tract after surgery, but it may also be needed permanently if large sections of the intestine have been removed. When a patient is dependent on the catheter for delivery of all nutrients, the procedure is termed total parenteral nutrition (TPN).

Managing feeding by tube or by catheter at home demands rigorous standards of care and cleanliness. Because patients with nasogastric tubes usually breathe through the mouth, they may need help in the form of wet swabs or frozen fruit juice cubes to moisten dried-out lips and mucous membranes. Chewing sugarless gum may stimulate the flow of saliva and provide some oral satisfaction.

Although many technical improvements have made procedures easier and more tolerable than in the past, patients on long-term tube feeding often experience a sense of withdrawal and depression. Counseling may help to smooth the initial adjustment, but most people eventually adapt well, focusing on the return to health instead of the relative inconvenience of tube feeding.

FEEDING SICK CHILDREN

Children's needs are more complicated than those of adults during illness. A diet has to provide sufficient nutrients and calories to maintain a healthy growth rate while also supplying the energy needed to fight the illness.

A sick child may need special help with feeding; finger foods and covered drinks with straws are much easier to manage than a tray laden with cutlery and spillable glassware. When the appetite is poor, parents or hospital caregivers may find it necessary to take the initiative by offering tempting foods and urging a listless young patient to take fluids and nourishment. However, it doesn't help to insist on a clean plate; most children will take as much as they can when they're ready. What is key is that an appealing, healthful selection of foods and beverages be available. Hospitals will frequently allow parents to bring a child's favorite foods from home.

FOOD PRESENTATION

It's important to take care in the presentation of food to an invalid. A weak appetite may be stimulated by the visual appeal of small, colorful portions attractively garnished and served at the correct temperature. Prepare textures that offer a pleasing contrast without taxing the patient's physical limitations (an elderly person, for example, may have difficulty chewing). Cut foods into manageable portions. A flower in a bud vase or juice served in a pretty glass may do more than any medication to lift the spirits and put the patient back on the road to health.

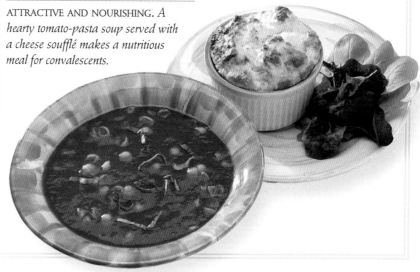

ATTRACTIVE AND NOURISHING. *A hearty tomato-pasta soup served with a cheese soufflé makes a nutritious meal for convalescents.*

HYPERACTIVITY

CONSUME
- *A variety of foods to provide a nutritionally complete diet.*

CUT DOWN ON
- *Caffeinated beverages.*
- *Hot dogs and other foods that contain large amounts of food additives and preservatives.*

AVOID
- *Self-treatment with high-dose vitamins and minerals.*
- *Diets that eliminate entire food groups.*

About 2 to 4 percent of all children suffer from hyperactivity (or attention deficit disorder), with boys outnumbering girls about fivefold. Parents often describe the hyperactive child as being in perpetual motion—always on the move, disruptive, impulsive, and unable to concentrate. Many researchers theorize that an imbalance in brain chemistry is responsible for the abnormal behavior, but a precise cause has not been identified.

In recent years, diet has been suggested as a possible cause of hyperactivity—a claim discounted by many experts. Although some nutritional deficiencies can affect behavior, these almost never occur in industrialized countries, where malnutrition is seldom a problem. Also, dozens of studies have failed to prove that diet plays any role in hyperactivity. Still, many parents and even some physicians believe that, at least for some children, there is a link. The diet hypothesis was first proposed in 1973 by Benjamin Feingold, a California allergist, who blamed hyperactivity on sensitivity to certain food additives and salicylates, compounds found in fruits, some vegetables, and in aspirin. Dr. Feingold recommended eliminating all foods that contain certain preservatives and artificial flavors and colors, as well as any natural sources of salicylates. Half of his hyperactive patients improved on this diet, and soon many doctors and parent groups were supporting the Feingold diet.

Although some reports suggest that an additive-free diet helps a few children, Dr. Feingold's finding of marked improvement in a significant percentage of cases has not been duplicated in scientific studies. Some pediatricians advise parents to try eliminating foods that are especially high in preservatives, dyes, and other additives—for example, hot dogs and other processed meats and some commercial baked goods—to see if there is an improvement. But avoiding all foods that contain natural salicylates is more problematic; there is no evidence that this actually helps, and it can lead to deficiencies of vitamin C, beta carotene, and other nutrients.

Caffeine has been linked to hyperactivity. Experts doubt that it actually causes the problem, but it may add to the restlessness of a hyperactive child. In any event, eliminating caffeine from a child's diet won't hurt.

Some proponents of orthomolecular therapy—the use of markedly high doses of vitamins and minerals to treat behavioral and other problems—advocate them as a treatment for hyperactivity. There is no evidence that this helps, but self-treating with megadose vitamins and minerals can cause serious nutritional imbalances and toxicity.

SUGAR CLEARED

Hyperactivity has often been blamed on a high intake of sugar. Again, there is no scientific proof of this. In fact, one study conducted by the National Institute of Mental Health in the U.S. found that children given a sugary drink were less active than a control group who had sugar-free drinks. Some researchers theorize that this calming effect is related to the fact that sugar prompts the brain to increase the production of serotonin, a chemical that reduces the brain's electrical activity. Even so, this is not a good reason to consume lots of sweets—sugar provides calories but is devoid of other nutrients; it also promotes dental disorders.

HYPOGLYCEMIA

CONSUME
- *Small meals that provide a balance of protein, carbohydrates, and fats.*

CUT DOWN ON
- *Carbohydrate-only (especially sugary) meals and snacks.*

AVOID
- *Consuming alcohol without food.*

Glucose, or blood sugar, is the body's major source of energy; it's also the only form of energy that the brain can use effectively. During digestion and metabolism, the liver converts all of the carbohydrates and about half of the protein in a meal into glucose, which is released into the bloodstream. In response to rising blood glucose levels, the pancreas secretes extra insulin, the hormone that enables cells to use the sugar to produce energy.

Low blood sugar, or hypoglycemia, occurs when the amount of insulin in the blood exceeds what is needed to metabolize the available glucose. It is seen often when a person with diabetes takes too much insulin, but it can also develop in other circumstances, such as an overconsumption of alcohol; taking large amounts of aspirin or acetaminophen, beta blockers, and some antipsychotic drugs; or when tumors develop that secrete insulin.

REACTIVE HYPOGLYCEMIA

An unusual condition known as reactive hypoglycemia occurs when the body secretes more insulin than it needs, causing a drop in blood glucose levels. Stress, missed meals, and a low-calorie diet of mostly carbohydrates can cause this type of hypoglycemia. Symptoms include dizziness, headache, hunger, trembling, palpitations, irritability, and mood swings. (A diabetic who takes an overdose of insulin has similar but more pronounced symptoms.)

Many people who experience vague, unexplained symptoms assume that they have reactive hypoglycemia, but the condition is rare and exists under very unusual circumstances. This is because the human body has a very sensitive feedback system that controls insulin secretion. Reactive hypoglycemia can only be diagnosed by monitoring blood glucose levels after ingestion of a known dose of glucose.

A low-calorie diet that is made up mostly of carbohydrates may produce mild symptoms of hypoglycemia even though the blood sugar levels are usually in the low-normal range. Here's what happens: The person may skip breakfast or have only simple carbohydrates—for example, a glass of orange juice and a sweet roll. The pancreas will secrete a fair amount of insulin to process the glucose in this meal, but since it contains no protein or fat, which are metabolized more slowly than carbohydrates, the body will burn the glucose in 2 or 3 hours. Sensing a need for more energy, the brain sends out powerful hunger signals; the person may also have a headache or feel dizzy. A sweet snack will satisfy this hunger and provide a quick burst of energy, but again, the pancreas will pump out enough insulin to quickly metabolize the glucose. If the scenario is repeated throughout the day, a pattern is established in which a person experiences symptoms that are temporarily alleviated by taking in more carbohydrates. The cycle can be broken by consuming regular meals that include small amounts of protein and fats along with starches. These take longer than sugars to be digested and converted into glucose, and allow for a steady release of energy.

INSULIN OVERDOSE

A much more serious type of hypoglycemia occurs when a diabetic takes more insulin than is needed to metabolize the available glucose. Many circumstances can affect the amount of insulin a diabetic requires: exercise, stress, infection, a skipped or late meal, even the weather. The onset of symptoms of an insulin reaction—hunger, tingling sensations, sweating, faintness, impaired vision, mood changes, palpitations, and a cold, clammy sensation—can be reversed by immediately eating a tablespoonful of sugar or honey, sucking on a hard candy, or drinking a glass of orange juice or sugary drink. If ignored, an insulin reaction can lead to coma and even death.

Case Study

Almost daily, Sally, a 39-year-old editor and vegetarian, experienced strange symptoms, which began with a nagging headache accompanied by dizziness, difficulty concentrating, a racing pulse, and severe hunger pangs. Taking a couple of aspirins and eating a candy bar alleviated her symptoms for a while, but in an hour or two, they'd return worse than before. At first Sally attributed her symptoms to job-related stress, but she worried that they reflected a disease.

A checkup failed to find abnormalities. Sally consulted still another doctor, who also found nothing wrong. Then she read an article that described her symptoms and provided a diagnosis: hypoglycemia.

Sally returned to her doctor and requested an oral glucose tolerance test—an examination that measures blood sugar levels after sugar consumption. The doctor, who had a number of patients with similar symptoms, assured Sally that she did not have true hypoglycemia.

Suspecting diet as the culprit, the doctor asked Sally to keep a diary of all the food she ate and any symptoms. The diary showed a familiar pattern— orange juice and coffee for breakfast, frequent snacks of candy or other sweets, a light lunch of a salad and an apple, and a low-fat vegetarian dinner with a glass or two of wine. The doctor explained that Sally's symptoms were brought on by an unbalanced diet. She urged Sally to start the day with more protein — perhaps a boiled egg and a glass of milk—and to have some yogurt or a sandwich for her mid-morning snack. Lunch could be a cup of lentil soup and a whole-grain pita filled with fresh vegetables and sprouts, and dinner a combination of grains and legumes for protein and starch. After a few weeks on this diet, Sally reported that her troubling symptoms had ceased.

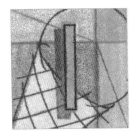

ICE CREAM

BENEFITS

- *A good source of calcium.*
- *Provides protein and digestible, high-calorie nutrition during an illness.*

DRAWBACKS

- *High in saturated fat and sugar.*

Federal standards decree that ice cream must be made with a minimum of 10 percent cream, or milk fat, and 36 percent solids (fat with protein, minerals, and lactose). Manufacturers may add various other ingredients, as well as enough air to double its volume. In general, the least expensive ice creams contain the minimum 10 percent fat and the maximum air, while the premium commercial brands have double the fat and half the air.

It is fat that gives ice cream its smooth texture; manufacturers of non-fat and low-fat ices and frozen yogurts compensate for the lack of fat by increasing the sugar—by up to twice the amount—and beating in less air. Therefore, although these products contain less fat, in the end they are not necessarily lower in calories.

Both soft ice cream and ice milk are 3 to 6 percent fat and 30 to 50 percent air. Sherbets are usually made with a small amount of milk fat and milk solids or, sometimes, egg white. Fruit ices, on the other hand, tend to be made with fruit pulp or juice, sugar, and water, with the possible addition

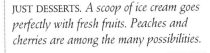

JUST DESSERTS. *A scoop of ice cream goes perfectly with fresh fruits. Peaches and cherries are among the many possibilities.*

of pectin or ascorbic acid. Most of these products contain about 200 calories per cup. Even a half cup of fat-free frozen yogurt with artificial sweetener has about 80 calories.

Ice cream has substantial amounts of calcium and protein, as well as some vitamin A and riboflavin. The price for these useful nutrients, however, is a large helping of saturated fat, with its adverse implications for heart disease, certain cancers, and other conditions. Fruit sorbets—which are high in sugar but fat-free—are a better choice when you want to end a meal with a frozen dessert. Fat-free frozen yogurt is a good substitute for ice cream; a half cup topped with fresh fruit and toasted wheat germ can satisfy cravings for a frosty treat and supply useful amounts of calcium, vitamins, and fiber.

WHAT'S IN A ½-CUP SERVING OF FROZEN DESSERT

TYPE	ENERGY (CALORIES)	FAT (g)	PROTEIN (g)	CARBOHYDRATE (g)	CALCIUM (mg)
Ice cream, vanilla	180	12	2	16	76
Ice cream, flavored	125–150*	6–8	2–3	16	73–93*
Ice milk, vanilla	90	3	2	15	88
Ice milk, chocolate	100	3	3	16	112
Fruit ice, sorbet	123	0	Tr	30	0
Frozen yogurt, fat-free	80	0	4	16	79
Sherbet, orange, made with milk fat and solids	135	2	1	29	52

* Varies according to flavor.

THE IMMUNE SYSTEM

The immune system defends the body from invasion and remembers every enemy it meets. Vitamins, minerals, and proteins help keep this defense system on the alert.

The immune system defends us against threats from both outside and inside the body. Most often, the external threats are infections caused by invading bacteria, viruses, and fungi, while abnormal or cancerous cells pose the major internal threats. In addition, this complex system oversees the repair of tissues that are injured by wounds or disease.

Once in a while the immune system mistakes a harmless foreign substance for an enemy, resulting in an allergic reaction, such as hives, hay fever, and asthma. Less commonly the immune system—mistaking an internal signal—attacks normal body tissue, leading to an autoimmune disease, such as diabetes, some types of arthritis, and lupus.

The most remarkable characteristic of the immune system is its "memory" for every foreign protein it encounters. Confronted with a virus or other invading organism, the system creates an antibody that will recognize it and mount an attack against it at any future encounter. This mechanism, called acquired immunity, is what makes vaccinations work.

SYSTEM FAILURE

Infection, cancer, and other illnesses develop when the immune system is overwhelmed or weakened by any number of stressors, including viruses and other invading organisms, malnutrition, and the consequences of

---

EAT PLENTY OF

- *Fruits and leafy vegetables for vitamins A and C; wheat germ and fortified cereals for vitamin E.*
- *Fatty fish and vegetable oils for omega-3 and omega-6 fatty acids.*
- *Shellfish, low-fat red meat, fortified whole-wheat breads and cereals, and legumes for protein, zinc, and iron.*

AVOID

- *Immune-power diets, which have no proven benefits.*

---

aging. Fortunately, antibiotics and sulfa drugs can wipe out most bacterial infections in otherwise healthy people; progress is also being made in the development of antiviral drugs. At times doctors purposely lower immunity to treat an autoimmune disease or prevent rejection of a donor organ.

DIETARY INFLUENCES

Proteins are central to the proper functioning of the immune system; antibodies are formed from various amino acids, especially arginine and glutamine. These amino acids are found in meat and other high-protein foods; the body can also manufacture them.

Omega-3 and omega-6 fatty acids, known to be beneficial in heart disease and other conditions, also seem to fight infection, although it's not clear how they work. Omega-3 fatty acids are especially beneficial in controlling inflammation and the harmful effects of rheumatoid arthritis and other autoimmune disorders.

ANTIOXIDANTS are also important to immune function: Vitamin A aids in warding off infection; vitamin E helps to preserve fatty acids; and vitamin C assists in bonding cells and strengthening the blood vessel walls.

Zinc and iron are among the minerals thought to boost immunity. A deficiency of zinc has been associated with slow wound healing, while adequate iron ensures that cells get the oxygen they need to function properly and resist disease. Both minerals are found in lean meat, poultry, shellfish, fortified whole-grain breads and cereals, and legumes.

FAD DIETS

Some unscrupulous practitioners, including opportunistic physicians, exploit the importance of the immune system and the difficulty of understanding its complexity by publicizing methods to boost your "immune power." These practitioners recommend a two-part remedial program, starting with an elimination diet, supposedly to "cleanse" the body, followed by megadoses of vitamins, minerals, and amino acids, supposedly to restore immune power. In reality, there is no evidence that such regimens boost immunity, and the high-dose supplements can be dangerous.

MINERALS

*The human body needs numerous minerals to carry out
its many vital functions. Luckily, most are required in tiny
amounts that are easily obtained from a balanced diet.*

Minerals are those elements that remain largely as ash when animal or plant tissues are burned. They constitute about 4 percent of our body weight and perform a variety of functions. To date, nutrition scientists have identified 16 minerals that are essential to maintain good health and promote proper metabolism and other bodily functions in humans. Calcium and a few others are present in relatively large amounts and are classified as macrominerals. However, most minerals are classified as trace, or micro, because they are needed in only minute amounts. The electrolytes generate electrical impulses to transport nerve messages; they also maintain the proper balances of fluids and body chemicals.

A varied and balanced diet provides all the essential minerals; supplements are generally not recommended, because many are highly toxic if consumed in large amounts. There are a few exceptions—for example, during pregnancy, when extra iron and calcium are needed. Also, the mineral content of foods varies according to the composition of the soil where the plants are grown or animals are grazed. Therefore, people may need dietary supplements in areas where the soil is deficient in a particular mineral.

A number of factors influence the body's ability to absorb and metabolize minerals. In general, the body is more efficient in absorbing a mineral during periods of increased need; thus,

---

BENEFITS
- *Build strong bones and teeth.*
- *Work with vitamins and enzymes to carry out many metabolic processes.*
- *Maintain the proper balance of body fluids and chemicals.*
- *Promote the proper function of most body systems.*

DRAWBACKS
- *Can be highly toxic if excessive amounts are consumed.*

---

a person who is anemic will absorb more iron from the diet than an individual who has a normal reserve of the mineral. Bran and other types of dietary fiber bind with some minerals to reduce absorption; in contrast, vitamin C increases the uptake of iron, calcium, and some other minerals.

THE MACROMINERALS
Minerals make up about 3 to 5 percent of normal body weight; most of this comes from the macrominerals that are stored in the bones. But minerals also circulate in the blood.

Calcium. The most abundant mineral in the body, calcium weighs in at 980 to 1,260g in the typical adult male, compared to only 760 to 900g for women. Because calcium is essential for building and maintaining strong bones and teeth, it's not surprising that these structures hold 99 percent of the

body's calcium. This mineral also ensures proper nerve and muscle function as it moves in and out of bone tissue and circulates through the body.

Milk, cheese, yogurt, and other milk products are the best sources of calcium; the mineral is also found in canned sardines and salmon (if the bones are eaten), tofu (soybean curd), broccoli, and a variety of other vegetables and fruits. In general, the calcium in milk or soft bones is easier to absorb than that in plant foods.

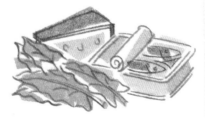

Calcium deficiency can cause rickets in children and osteomalacia, a disorder characterized by soft, aching bones, in adults. In some cases, calcium deficiency is due to a lack of vitamin D, which the body requires to absorb the mineral. The deficiency may also be a result of physical inactivity, especially complete bed rest, which increases calcium loss. In addition, women need estrogen, the major female sex hormone, to metabolize calcium, which is why older women are so vulnerable to osteoporosis.

Magnesium. The body contains only about 28g of magnesium, 60 percent of which is stored in the bones; the rest circulates in the blood or is stored in muscle tissue. Magnesium is essential to build bones and is needed for proper muscle function, energy metabolism, to transmit nerve impulses, and to make genetic material and protein.

Because magnesium is found in so many foods—green leafy vegetables, grains, legumes, meat, poultry, fish, and eggs—deficiency is rare. Reserves can be depleted, however, by alcoholism, prolonged diarrhea, liver or kidney disease, and severe diabetes.

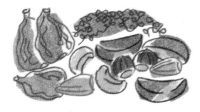

Phosphorus. The second most plentiful mineral in the body, phosphorus works in conjunction with calcium and fluoride to give bones and teeth their strength and hardness. On average, it makes up 1 percent of normal body weight; 85 percent of this is in the bones, and the remainder is found in soft tissue. Phosphorus is essential for many metabolic processes and the storage and release of energy, as well as the activation of the B-complex vitamins and many enzymes.

Foods that are high in calcium (see facing page) also tend to be high in phosphorus; other good sources include meat, whole-grain products, and soft drinks.

THE TRACE MINERALS

Only very small, or trace, amounts of the following minerals are required to meet normal body requirements.

Chromium. Insulin and chromium appear to act together to metabolize glucose, the body's major fuel. Brewer's yeast is very high in chromium; other good sources include wheat germ, whole-grain products, liver, cheese, beer, and molasses.

Copper. A component of many enzymes, copper is essential for making red blood cells, skin pigment, connective tissue, and nerve fibers; it also stimulates absorption of iron. Excessive zinc appears to reduce the body's ability to absorb and store copper. Copper deficiency results in anemia, deterioration of the heart muscle, inelastic blood vessels, various skeletal defects, nerve degeneration, skin and hair abnormalities, and infertility.

Liver is the richest source of copper, but the mineral is also found in seafood, legumes, nuts and seeds, prunes, and barley. Using unlined copper pans can result in copper toxicity. Excessive copper can cause severe liver disease and mental deterioration; several metabolic disorders can cause a buildup of copper in the liver and other tissues. Patients suffering from Wilson's disease, for example, must take drugs to eliminate copper from their body.

Fluoride. Best known for preventing cavities and other dental disorders, fluoride is also needed to maintain strong bones. Fluoride occurs naturally in some areas; in fact, it was in these regions that the relationship between decreased incidence of tooth decay and fluoride was first noted. Some groups oppose adding fluoride to drinking

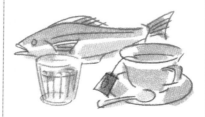

water, claiming it is a carcinogen. The prevailing scientific opinion, however, is that fluoridating drinking water is an appropriate health measure.

Iodine. This mineral has only one known function in humans: it is necessary to make thyroid hormones. An iodine deficiency can result in an overgrown thyroid gland, or goiter; in some severe cases, it can lead to hypo-

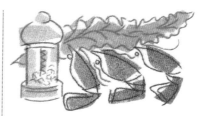

thyroidism. In addition, a baby borne by a woman with iodine deficiency may develop cretinism, a devastating type of mental retardation.

Seafood, kelp, and vegetables grown in iodine-rich soil are good sources of the mineral. Iodized salt is advisable in areas where the soil lacks iodine.

Iron. The body has only 3g to 5g of iron, 75 percent of which is in hemoglobin, the pigment in red blood cells that carries oxygen. Iron-deficiency ANEMIA is the most common nutritional deficiency in developed countries, but most cases are due to chronic blood loss, not an iron-poor diet. There are two types of iron: Heme is found in meat, poultry, fish, and eggs; nonheme is also found in animal products, as well as in vegetables, fruits, juices, grains, and fortified cereals. About 20 to 30 percent of heme iron is absorbed; lesser amounts of nonheme iron are absorbed, depending upon need and other dietary factors. Consuming nonheme iron with vitamin C or meat increases its absorption; bran, the tannins in tea, phytates in grains, and oxalates in many foods reduce its absorption.

As the body breaks down old red blood cells, it recycles most of their iron. A healthy adult man loses about 1mg of iron per day; compared to 1.5mg per day in a woman who is still menstruating. Except for pregnant women, the typical Canadian diet provides ample amounts of iron.

Manganese. A component of numerous enzymes, manganese plays an important role in metabolism; it is also needed to build bones and tendons. Manganese deficiency is unknown in humans, largely because most plant foods contain small amounts.

MINERAL	BEST FOOD SOURCES	ROLE IN HEALTH
MACROMINERALS		
Calcium	Milk and milk products; tofu; canned sardines and salmon (including bones); dark green vegetables.	Builds strong bones and teeth; vital to muscle and nerve function, blood clotting, and metabolism.
Magnesium	Leafy green vegetables; legumes and whole-grain cereals and breads; meats, poultry, fish, and eggs.	Stimulates bone growth; necessary for muscle function and metabolism.
Phosphorus	Meat, poultry, fish, egg yolks, legumes, dairy products, soft drinks.	Helps maintain strong bones and teeth; component of some enzymes; essential for proper metabolism.
MICROMINERALS		
Chromium	Brewer's yeast, whole-grain products, liver, cheese, beer.	Works with insulin to metabolize glucose.
Copper	Liver, shellfish, legumes, nuts, prunes.	Promotes iron absorption; essential to red blood cells, connective tissue, nerve fibers, and skin pigment. Component of several enzymes.
Fluoride	Fluoridated water; tea.	Helps maintain strong bones and teeth.
Iodine	Iodized salt, seafood, foods grown in iodine-rich soil.	Necessary to make thyroid hormones.
Iron	Liver, meat, seafood, legumes, fortified cereals.	Needed for transport and storage of oxygen.
Manganese	Coffee, tea, nuts, legumes, bran.	Component of many enzymes needed for metabolism; necessary for bone and tendon formation.
Molybdenum	Liver and other organ meats; dark green leafy vegetables; whole-grain products.	Component of enzymes needed for metabolism; instrumental in iron storage.
Selenium	Poultry, seafood, organ meats, whole-grain products, onions, garlic, mushrooms.	Antioxidant that works with vitamin E to protect cell membranes from oxidative damage.
Sulfur	Protein foods.	Component of two essential amino acids.
Zinc	Oysters, meat, yogurt, fortified cereals.	Instrumental in metabolic action of enzymes; essential for growth and reproduction.
ELECTROLYTES		
Chloride	Table salt, seafood, milk, eggs, meat.	Maintains proper body chemistry. Used to make digestive juices.
Potassium	Avocados, bananas, citrus and dried fruits; legumes and many vegetables; whole-grain products.	Along with sodium, helps to maintain fluid balance; promotes proper metabolism and muscle function.
Sodium	Table salt, dairy products, seafood, seasonings, most processed foods.	With potassium, regulates the body's fluid balance; promotes proper muscle function.

*Based on the Nutrition Research Division of Health and Welfare Canada Recommended Nutrient Intakes (RNIs).

**Many experts recommend 1,000 to 1,500mg following menopause.

RECOMMENDED NUTRIENT INTAKES* (FOR ADULTS OVER 24)		SYMPTOMS OF DEFICIENCY	SYMPTOMS OF EXCESS
MALES	FEMALES		
800mg	800mg**	Rickets in children; easy fractures, brittle bones, and osteoporosis in adults.	Calcium deposits in body tissues; abdominal pain. Inhibits iron absorption.
250mg	200mg	Lethargy, cramps, muscle weakness, cardiac arrhythmias.	Diarrhea.
1,000mg	850mg	Weakness and bone pain. Deficiency is rare.	Decreased blood calcium.
0.05–0.2mg***	0.05–0.2mg***	Diabeteslike symptoms.	Unknown for dietary chromium. Chromium salt is toxic.
2–3mg***	2–3mg***	Anemia marked by abnormal development of bones, nerves, lungs, and hair color.	Vomiting, diarrhea, and liver disease.
1.5–4mg***	1.5–4mg***	Tooth decay.	Mottling of tooth enamel.
160mcg	160mcg	Goiter; cretinism in babies.	Abnormal thyroid function.
9mg	9–13mg	Iron-deficiency anemia.	Organ damage, especially liver and heart.
2.5–5mg***	2.5–5mg***	Unknown.	Nerve damage.
75–250mcg***	75–250mcg***	Unknown.	Goutlike joint pain.
70mcg	55mcg	Heart disease and rare form of anemia.	Diarrhea, nausea, abdominal pain, tooth damage, fatigue, irritability, hair and nail loss.
Not established	Not established	Unknown.	None with dietary sulfur.
12mg	9mg	Low immunity; slow healing of wounds; retarded growth and sexual development.	Nausea, vomiting, heart muscle damage, kidney failure, muscle pain, atherosclerosis.
2–5g***	2–5g***	Deficiency is extremely rare; causes upset in acid-base balance when it occurs.	Disturbance in body chemistry.
2–6g***	2–6g***	Muscle weakness; cardiac arrhythmias.	Nausea and diarrhea; potentially fatal cardiac arrhythmias.
1–3g***	1–3g***	Muscle cramps, headaches, and weakness; rare, except as a result of injury or illness.	Exacerbates hypertension, heart failure, and kidney disease.

*** Recommended Nutrient Intakes (RNIs) have not been established; values for these minerals are based on current expert opinion.

Molybdenum. Another component of many enzymes, molybdenum helps regulate iron storage and is instrumental in the production of uric acid. A deficiency of this mineral almost never occurs. Overdoses, which cause goutlike joint symptoms, are also rare but have been reported in some parts of Armenia, where the soil is rich in this mineral.

Selenium. An important ANTIOXIDANT, selenium interacts with vitamin E to prevent the free radicals produced during oxygen metabolism from damaging body fat and other tissues. Human selenium deficiency is rare except in areas where the soil contains little of the mineral, where it causes a rare type of heart disease in children.

Foods that are high in selenium include seafood, organ meats, poultry, whole-grain products, mushrooms, onions, and garlic. Recent reports that selenium may help prevent cancer have not been proved, but they have led to increased sales of selenium supplements. Although selenium toxicity is uncommon, there have been a few cases among people taking high doses. Symptoms include nausea, diarrhea, fatigue, damage to the skin and nerves, and loss of hair and nails.

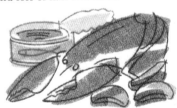

Sulfur. A component of several amino acids and B vitamins, sulfur is found in every cell of the body; it is particularly concentrated in the skin, nails, and hair. Humans cannot develop a sulfur deficiency, nor is it possible to overdose on dietary sulfur. However, some inorganic sulfur salts are toxic, and others, such as the sulfites used as food preservatives, can trigger asthma attacks and other allergic reactions in susceptible people.

Zinc. An essential component of many enzymes, zinc is necessary for some metabolic processes, normal growth and sexual development, and proper immune system function. It is also needed to make genetic materials (DNA and RNA) and for proper wound healing. A deficiency results in increased susceptibility to infection, fatigue, lethargy, loss of appetite, balding, and taste abnormalities.

Zinc is found in many foods; especially good sources include beef and other meats, eggs, oysters and other seafood, yogurt, wheat germ, and fortified cereals. The phytates in bran and some whole-grain products, however, bind with zinc and prevent the body from absorbing it. Even so, zinc deficiency is rare in North America.

In recent years zinc supplements have been promoted to increase immunity. These should be used only when specifically recommended by a doctor, however, because too much zinc can cause diarrhea, vomiting, degeneration of the heart muscle, accelerated development of atherosclerosis, kidney failure, and bleeding, among many other symptoms.

THE ELECTROLYTES

Three essential minerals are classified as electrolytes, substances that dissociate into ions when placed in water or other fluids. In the human body electrolytes conduct electrical charges and are instrumental in nerve and muscle function; they also help maintain the proper balance of body fluids.

Chloride. A component of table salt, chloride is essential to maintain the body's proper acid-base balance. Chloride is also a component of hydrochloric acid, one of the digestive juices produced in the stomach. A diet that includes a moderate amount of salt provides adequate chloride; deficiencies are rare but may occur during periods of excessive sweating or prolonged vomiting or diarrhea.

Potassium. Along with sodium, potassium helps regulate the body's balance of fluids. Potassium is essential for many metabolic processes; it is also instrumental in the transmission of nerve impulses, proper muscle function, and maintaining normal blood pressure. Most plant foods contribute varying amounts of potassium; especially rich sources include dried fruits, bananas, tomatoes, citrus fruits, avocados, potatoes, green vegetables, legumes, whole grains, and nuts.

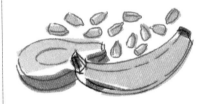

Prolonged diarrhea or the use of diuretics to treat high blood pressure can lead to a potassium deficiency; typical symptoms include an irregular heartbeat, muscle weakness, and irritability. Caution is necessary when taking potassium supplements, however; an overdose can cause nausea, diarrhea, and serious cardiac arrhythmias that can result in sudden death.

Sodium. Table salt is composed of sodium and chloride, and the terms salt and sodium are often used interchangeably. Sodium is found in all body fluids and is largely responsible for determining the body's total water content. Like potassium, sodium ions carry positive electrical charges and help regulate nerve and muscle function. These two electrolytes also maintain the fluid balance inside and outside of body cells.

A sodium deficiency is very rare; overconsumption is a much more common problem, especially among those who liberally salt their food. In susceptible people excessive salt is linked to high blood pressure; it can also cause swollen ankles and fingers and other signs of a buildup of body fluids, or edema.

MONONUCLEOSIS

CONSUME PLENTY OF
- *Fruit and vegetable juices for vitamins and minerals.*
- *Milk shakes for calories, minerals, and vitamin D.*
- *Soups for energy and fiber.*
- *Soft foods to soothe a sore throat.*

AVOID
- *Alcohol.*

A common disease, mononucleosis is caused by the Epstein-Barr virus, which infects at least half of all Canadian children by the age of 5. The majority of these infections pass unrecognized, because the symptoms of mild fever and slight fatigue last only a short time and resolve spontaneously. The Epstein-Barr virus is transmitted in the saliva by coughing, sneezing, or kissing. Otherwise, most people who have only casual contact with an infected person do not get the disease.

Mononucleosis causes more debilitating illness in adolescents and adults, who generally have fatigue, fever, severe sore throat, and swollen lymph nodes. Patients usually lose their appetite and complain of headaches and general achiness. Often, the fever and sore throat are misdiagnosed as tonsillitis. If the sore throat is treated with ampicillin, an antibiotic similar to penicillin, the patient with mononucleosis develops a rash. The spleen—and, less often, the liver—may become enlarged. In very severe cases the patient may develop jaundice.

The symptoms typically last for a week or two, and most people are able to return to work at that time. In a few cases, however, recovery may take several months, as a low-grade fever, poor appetite, and fatigue persist for weeks after the other symptoms have disappeared. When this happens, mononucleosis may be mistaken for chronic fatigue syndrome. In the past, chronic fatigue syndrome was at times referred to as chronic Epstein-Barr infection, but it is now known that they are unrelated.

THE ROLE OF DIET
A well-balanced diet can aid in recovery and boost the strength of the IMMUNE SYSTEM to fight mononucleosis. Stimulate a poor appetite with several light, appetizing meals rather than a few larger ones, which may be daunting. During the acute phase, when fever may be high, it's important to drink plenty of liquids in order to prevent dehydration. Drink at least eight glasses of water or juice daily. During recuperation, juices have the added benefit of providing vitamins and other immune-boosting nutrients.

Milk shakes and fruit nectars diluted with water soothe a sore throat and provide calories for energy, along with minerals and vitamins. Applesauce and other stewed fruits supply soluble fiber, which helps prevent constipation. Soups are nutritious and easy to eat. Soft foods, such as puddings, scrambled eggs, cottage cheese, and yogurt, are easily swallowed, even by someone with a sore throat. Fruits and vegetables can be pureed to make them easier to swallow; serve vegetables as a sauce over complex carbohydrates, such as rice or soft noodles. Herbal teas are soothing, and gargling with tepid salt water can relieve a sore throat. Avoid alcohol, which weakens the immune system and can further damage the liver.

TREATMENT
See a physician if you think you have mononucleosis, since blood tests are necessary for a definitive diagnosis. Rest is an important part of recovery. Take aspirin or some other nonsteroidal anti-inflammatory drug (NSAID) to ease symptoms. However, since the disease is a viral and not a bacterial infection, it should not be treated with antibiotics. People with mononucleosis just have to wait it out. Long-term complications are rare, but activity should be limited until you feel strength returning. Don't engage in vigorous activity until the doctor says the spleen has returned to its normal size; abrupt force can rupture an enlarged spleen and cause serious problems.

Case Study

When 16-year-old Todd became ill with severe fatigue and swollen glands, his mother feared that he might have leukemia. After a doctor's visit she was understandably relieved when blood tests found he had mononucleosis instead. But she became increasingly concerned when 6 weeks later, he still lacked energy and only picked at his meals.

A dietitian advised Todd's mother to try giving him smaller, frequent snacks of his favorite foods, such as milk shakes, scrambled eggs, puddings, pizza topped with cheese and vegetables, hearty soups, and ample fruit juices and nectars. This approach seemed to work, and before long Todd made a full recovery.

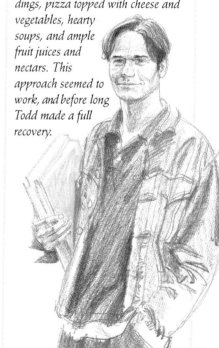

PREPARATION AND STORAGE OF FOOD

*The techniques used to clean, store, and prepare food not only
affect its taste, texture, and nutritional value, but are also
instrumental in preventing spoilage and food-borne illness.*

By using the proper methods to prepare and store foods, you can keep them wholesome and nutritious; preserve their appetizing appearance, taste, and texture; and use them economically. Exposure to heat, light, moisture, and air can cause some foods to spoil or deteriorate, and many lose flavor, texture, and nutritional value if kept too long. Improper handling and storage also raise the possibility of food poisoning.

FOOD STORAGE

Heat and humidity greatly increase the risk of food spoilage, so you should never store foods in warm places, such as near the stove or refrigerator or under the kitchen sink. To minimize the risk of contamination and accidental poisoning, always keep foodstuffs and cleaning products in separate areas.

Because even canned foods deteriorate with time, you should stack cans in the order of their date so that the oldest can is used first. Store them away from moisture in a 50°F to 70°F (10°C to 21°C) temperature range, preferably at the cooler end of the range. Dry goods should be kept in a cool, dark, dry pantry or cupboard and used before the expiration date.

GRAINS AND NUTS
Grains, flours, and other foods packed in materials easily penetrated by moths and other insects—for example, unopened cardboard boxes, paper bags, and cellophane packages—should be transferred to plastic, metal, or glass containers with tight-fitting lids. (Even then, insect eggs in the flour or grains may hatch. To kill the eggs before storage, put the product in a microwave oven set on High for 2 to 3 minutes; or refrigerate it to help prevent the eggs from hatching.) Whole-grain flours and meals spoil within a few weeks, because their fats turn rancid. Storing them in a freezer extends their shelf life.

Bread, cereals, and crackers are normally best kept in closed containers at room temperature. Cereals, like other foods made from grains, should be stored in a dark place, because they will lose riboflavin if left exposed to light. Yeast breads will keep for a few days if wrapped in plastic or foil and stored in a cool, dark place, such as a bread box. In hot weather, refrigeration may be required to prevent mold.

Unshelled nuts can be kept at room temperature for 3 to 6 months; shelled nuts may become rancid unless refrigerated or frozen. Discard any that smell musty or are moldy.

PRODUCE
Raw fruits and VEGETABLES often slowly lose their vitamins when kept at room temperature, but tropical fruits deteriorate rapidly if stored in the cold. Most produce is best stored at about 50°F (10°C); if refrigerated, put it in the crisper section; the restricted space slows down moisture loss. Avoid storing fruits and vegetables for long periods in sealed plastic bags; they cut off the air supply, causing the produce to rot. Paper and cellophane are better storage materials, because they are permeable. Keep juice in a small container so that vitamins are not lost through exposure to oxygen.

In regions where winter temperatures average 30°F (–1°C) or less, fruits and vegetables bought in bulk can be stored in a cool basement or root cellar. Carrots, cabbage, and lettuce keep well at about 32°F (0°C). Wash lettuce and other salad greens, spin dry, and store them in a plastic bag with a paper towel to absorb any excess moisture. To prevent rot caused by dampness during storage, wash other produce just before using them.

Leave the stems on berries until you're ready to use them, and refrigerate peas and beans in their pods. Cut the green tops off root vegetables, such as carrots, BEETS, parsnips, and turnips, or they will continue to draw nourishment from the roots.

When stored below 40°F (4°C), potatoes develop a sweetish taste from the conversion of starch to sugar; the sweetness disappears when the tubers are returned to room temperature. Potatoes are often packaged in burlap bags or covered with mesh that protects them from light while still allowing air to circulate. Store potatoes in the dark, because exposure to light causes poisonous alkaloids, such as solanine and chaconine, to form.

Freezing raw fruits and vegetables causes the water they contain to form ice crystals that break down cell membranes and walls, resulting in a mushy texture and a loss of nutrients. Deterioration of fruits and vegetables can also be caused by enzymatic activity; blanching prevents this problem. Immerse vegetables for a few seconds in rapidly boiling water to deactivate their enzymes, then plunge them into cold water to stop the cooking process. Most fruits are not suitable for blanching, but you can prevent browning and deterioration by packing them in a solution of sugar, either with or without ascorbic acid.

All produce should be wrapped airtight to prevent freezer burn, which causes dry patches that have a rough texture and "off" taste. Frozen vegetables should be cooked straight from the freezer; thawing encourages the destructive activity of residual enzymes and microorganisms. Do not refreeze foods that have been thawed.

The home canning process preserves foods by rapid heating of hermetically sealed containers. The heat destroys microorganisms and stops enzyme ac-

AIRTIGHT. *Fill food storage containers close to the brim, and remove as much air as possible before sealing storage bags.*

tion, and the vacuum seal prevents contamination. An improperly canned food may cause serious food poisoning with the potentially lethal *Clostridium botulinum.* Long boiling after opening the container will destroy the botulin toxins but not the spores, which can survive boiling for as long as 5 hours. Cans and jars that show any sign of bacterial activity—bubbles, incomplete seals, or escape of gas on opening—must be discarded.

Surprisingly, some commercially processed foods may be more nutritious than fresh. Produce for freezing or canning is often harvested in peak condition and processed quickly to preserve its appearance and nutritional value. Many fresh fruits and vegetables, on the other hand, are picked before ripening and matured under refrigeration; they never reach peak flavor. Look for vine- and tree-ripened varieties, and buy produce in season for economy, flavor, and nutrition.

MEAT, POULTRY, AND FISH

Store meats and fish in the coldest part of the refrigerator. Wrap meat for freezing in freezer paper. Avoid using gas-permeable plastic wrap; it allows moisture to evaporate and causes freezer burn. Shellfish cannot be kept more than a few hours at refrigerator temperature, but they last 2 or 3 days on ice or at a temperature below 32°F (0°C).

Hot dogs and cold cuts stay fresh until their expiration dates if they are refrigerated unopened in their original vacuum-sealed bags. Once opened, however, they should be rewrapped in an airtight bag and used within a few days. Cured and smoked meats are best stored in their original wrappings; make sure that cold cuts bought from the deli counter are wrapped well and used within a day or two. Meat with discoloration, an off smell, or any sign of mold must be discarded. The one exception to this rule is mold on dry salami; simply trim away the mold and the adjacent inch of meat. The unmoldy meat is still edible.

DAIRY PRODUCTS

Fresh milk and cream should be tightly sealed to prevent tainting by odors from other foods. Milk retains its nutritional value better in cartons than in clear bottles or plastic jugs, because exposure to light destroys some of the vitamin A and riboflavin. Store nonfat powdered milk in a tightly closed container at room temperature in a place where it's not exposed to light.

Keep soft cheese and butter tightly covered and refrigerated. Because of concerns about chemical contamination, some people keep plastic materials away from fatty foods, including cheese and butter. Foil is a good wrapper. Butter freezes well in its original wrapping. It's not necessary to refrigerate hard cheese and other ripened cheeses, which keep well covered in a cool, dark cupboard. If mold develops, pare it off; the cheese remains safe to eat.

OILS AND SUGARS

Fats turn rancid on exposure to air and pick up odors from other foods. Store tightly sealed oils in a dark cupboard or in the refrigerator. Exposure to light and warm temperatures can rob oils of vitamins A, D, and E. The cloudiness that forms in some oils when refrigerated will clear at room temperature.

Margarine, like butter, should be well covered and refrigerated; stores for future use may be frozen. You can refrigerate commercial mayonnaise after opening it. Use homemade mayonnaise as soon as it's made, however; discard leftovers to reduce the risk of food poisoning by salmonella bacteria.

Corn syrup and molasses keep well at room temperature, because they are too sugary for bacteria to thrive. However, natural maple syrup and artificially flavored syrups are susceptible to molds; refrigerate them after opening. Crystallized maple syrup, like honey, will liquefy if the bottle is warmed in a pan of water. Refrigerate opened jams and spreads.

FOOD PREPARATION

Cooking for too long or at too high a heat and using excessive liquids are common food preparation faults that detract from flavor and nutritional value. It is the water-soluble vitamins that are lost through poor preparation. Vitamin C is more easily destroyed than any other nutrient, so if vitamin C is conserved, others will be too.

MEATS AND FISH

Trim visible fat off red meat before cooking it to reduce calories, saturated fat, and traces of fat-soluble pollu-

tants. Discard poultry skin; it is high in saturated fat and calories. Make up for lost flavor with herbs and spices.

You can wipe red meat with a damp cloth or wash it to remove animal hairs or other contaminants. Wash poultry under running water and pat it dry with paper towels before preparation. Some experts recommend washing with diluted vinegar to reduce the risk of food poisoning from bacterial contamination. Rinse fish and pat dry.

Dry cooking methods—roasting, baking, broiling, and grilling—are suitable for tender cuts of meat. Moist-heat methods—poaching, braising, and stewing in liquid, such as stock or wine—break down the connective tissue in leaner, tougher cuts. Strain and rapidly boil down the liquid to make a nutrient-rich sauce.

A meat thermometer is useful for indicating if dry-cooked meat is done. A thermometer in a rare-cooked roast or broiled steak should register 140°F (60°C), the temperature at which most food-borne bacteria are killed. Ground meat is handled often, so it is very susceptible to contamination and should not be eaten rare; hamburgers should be brownish-pink to brown in the center. Poultry is cooked when the leg joints move easily and the juices run clear. Fish should flake easily with a fork when thoroughly cooked. Pork should have no pink color. Most cured hams are sold fully cooked and can be eaten cold or reheated.

FRUITS, VEGETABLES, AND GRAINS

If left to soak in water, vegetables lose vitamins and minerals. Right before using them, wash vegetables and fruits under running water to remove soil, insects, and water-soluble pesticides. Scrub heavily soiled produce or wax-treated citrus peels with just a little dish detergent and rinse thoroughly.

Most nutrients in produce are concentrated in the skin or immediately

below it. Unless fruits and vegetables were treated with wax coatings or pesticides, cook them in their skins and peel after boiling. The coarse outer leaves of many green vegetables have more concentrated nutrients than the hearts, but—unless organic or home-grown—they are also more exposed to pesticides and are better discarded.

Chopped and bruised fruits and vegetables rapidly lose vitamins A and C, because fluids drain out of broken tissues or deteriorate on exposure to the air. Cook fruits and vegetables whole or in large pieces, whenever possible, and do not chop, peel, or tear them until you're ready to cook them or prepare them for serving raw.

While most vegetables, including root vegetables, can be eaten raw, they are more often prepared by boiling, steaming, or frying. Steaming and stir-frying use little water, so they preserve nutritional content. When boiling vegetables, bring water to a boil first, then add the vegetables and cover with a tight-fitting lid. To add flavor and nutrients to soups and stews, recycle the drained cooking liquids.

Cooked vegetables should retain their crispness; overcooking makes them mushy and less nutritious. Some cooks add baking soda to preserve color, but this also destroys the nutritional content and breaks down the plant tissues, giving a slimy texture to green vegetables.

Commercially canned vegetables should be reheated but not recooked, which makes them soft. Home-canned vegetables, especially those low in acid, should be boiled for at least 10 minutes to destroy any bacteria.

Rice and pasta should never be washed, although rice (like other grains and legumes) should be picked over for pebbles and other contaminants. Measure the liquid for cooking rice and other grains; usually, twice the volume of liquid will be completely absorbed without the loss of nutrients.

HOW TO FREEZE AND THAW FOODS SAFELY

FOOD	PREPARA-TION	PACKAGING	TIPS	USE WITHIN (MONTHS)	THAWING (HOURS PER LB.)	
					REFRIGERATOR	ROOM TEMPERATURE
Apples	Sprinkle with lemon juice or powdered ascorbic acid.	Use plastic container or freezer bags.	Alternatively, freeze in syrup containing ascorbic acid.	9	6	3–4
Berries	Freeze on baking sheet; then pack in plastic bags. Freeze soft berries in sugar and syrup.	Transfer to a closed container.	Strawberries and raspberries may be frozen without sugar.	9	6	2
Peaches and plums	Remove pits. Wash and peel peaches. Pack with syrup and ascorbic acid to preserve color.	Use plastic containers or waxed cartons.	A tablespoon of lemon juice per pint of syrup preserves color.	9	6	3–4
Vegetables, green	Wash, trim, blanch, and drain.	Use plastic freezer bags or cartons.	Squeeze air out of bags.	12	6	3
Butter	Freeze in its wrapper.	Overwrap if it is soft.	Unsalted butter stores longer than salted.	3–8	3	1–2
Beef and lamb; pork roasts	Cut into meal-size portions.	Cover protruding bones with foil and wrap tightly with extra layers so that holes are not poked through the wrappings.	Debone joints before freezing to save freezer space.	9–12 (pork roasts, 9)	5	2
Ground meat	Divide into meal-size portions.	Use plastic containers or sealed freezer bags.	Freeze only fresh-ground meat.	4	6	1–2
Pork and lamb chops	Separate with sheets of freezer paper.	Wrap tightly in foil, not plastic.	Thaw pork or lamb chops in refrigerator.	6	3–5	2
Sausages (commercial)	None necessary.	Freeze in commercial packaging. Use freezer bags or plastic wrap for fresh sausages.	Cured and sliced meats do not keep as well as solid cuts.	1	3–5	1–2
Fish steaks	Separate into meal-size portions; wrap in freezer paper.	Wrap in plastic wrap, freezer paper, or foil.	Dry with paper towels to absorb moisture before freezing.	2	8	4
Fish, whole (white and oily)	Scale and fillet.	Wrap in plastic wrap, freezer paper, or foil.	Cut into meal-size portions before wrapping.	2	8	4

PROSTATE PROBLEMS

CONSUME PLENTY OF

- *Tomatoes, red grapefruits, watermelons, and berries for lycopene.*
- *Vegetable oils, margarine, wheat germ, whole-grain products, and nuts and seeds for vitamin E.*
- *Fruits and vegetables for antioxidants.*
- *Fish, shellfish, lean meat, yogurt, legumes, and other zinc-rich foods.*
- *Fluids to flush the bladder.*

CUT DOWN ON

- *Fatty foods, especially animal products.*

AVOID

- *Alcohol, caffeine, spicy foods, and other substances that irritate the urinary tract.*
- *Excessive weight gain.*

The prostate, a walnut-size gland located just below the bladder, is the source of many male urinary problems, including cancer, benign enlargement, and inflammation (prostatitis). Sexually transmitted diseases, urinary tract infections, and such lifestyle habits as smoking, heavy alcohol consumption, and a high-fat diet seem to predispose a man to some of these problems. But often, factors that are beyond our control are more instrumental.

As a man ages, the prostate gland tends to enlarge, a condition called benign prostatic hypertrophy, or BPH. About one-third of all men over 50 experience noncancerous enlargement of the prostate gland, the result of a gradual process that can eventually cause severe obstruction of urinary flow.

Prostate cancer, with an estimated 18,000 new cases a year, is the most common male malignancy. If it is treated in an early stage, this type of cancer is highly curable. In many cases, however, it has already spread to other organs at the time of diagnosis. For this

reason, the Canadian Cancer Society recommends that all men over 50 undergo annual screening for prostate cancer, starting with a digital rectal examination. The same group also advocates that a blood test to measure prostate-specific antigen (PSA), a possible indicator of cancer, should be done annually in addition to the rectal exam, starting at age 50.

The treatment of prostate disorders varies, depending on the underlying condition. Prostatitis is usually treated with antibiotics, warm baths, and occasionally prostatic massage. Some men with BPH require no treatment; other cases may call for surgery to remove the enlarged part of the prostate or drugs to shrink the gland. Prostate cancer may be treated with surgery, radiation, hormone therapy, or a combination of these methods.

THE ROLE OF DIET

Diet cannot cure prostate problems, but it may play a role in maintaining the health of the gland, and it may also help prevent prostate cancer. A recent study of nearly 48,000 men found that lycopene, a pigment that is found in such foods as tomatoes, red grapefruits, watermelons, and berries, appears to reduce the risk of prostate cancer. These findings support earlier recommendations to increase consumption of fruits and vegetables, which are high in other ANTIOXIDANTS and bioflavonoid pigments that protect against various cancers. Cooking appears to release more of the lycopene in tomatoes, so tomato-based pasta sauces and soups may be especially beneficial.

The human body needs zinc in order to use the lycopenes in foods. Zinc-rich foods include whole fish and shellfish (especially oysters), baked potatoes (if the skin is eaten), lean meat, calves' liver, yogurt, and legumes.

Vitamin E has also been associated with reducing inflammation and per-

HELPFUL FOODS

Tomatoes, watermelons, grapefruits, and berries for lycopene; have 10 servings a week.

Tofu and other soy products to help prevent prostate enlargement; consume 4 or 5 times a week.

Nuts, seeds, wheat germ, grains, and eggs for vitamin E; eat 1 or 2 servings daily.

Oysters, yogurt, and other foods high in zinc daily.

Fish and vegetable oils for daily allowance of polyunsaturated fats.

haps protecting against prostate cancer. Good sources include margarine, vegetable oils, egg yolks, nuts and seeds, wheat germ, and whole-grain products.

Tofu and other soy products appear to help prevent prostate enlargement. This effect is attributed to isoflavones, plant chemicals that help lower dihydrotestosterone (DHT), a male hormone that stimulates the overgrowth of prostate tissue. Some experts credit the large amount of soy products in the Japanese diet with their low incidence of prostate problems. The composition of fats in the diet also appears to play a role in prostate health. Fish and vegetable oils that are high in polyunsaturated fats seem to reduce the risk of prostate cancer. In contrast, a diet that is high in saturated animal fats, as well as obesity, has been linked to an increased incidence.

Anyone with an enlarged prostate should drink plenty of water and other nonalcoholic fluids. He should also eliminate from his diet caffeine and spicy foods that irritate the bladder.

PROTEIN: THE BODY-BUILDING NUTRIENT

*Every cell in the body needs protein for growth
and repair. Protein also plays an essential role in
digestion, immunity, and many other body functions.*

Protein is the quintessential nutrient that every cell in the human body requires for growth or repair. Also, the antibodies that protect us from disease, the enzymes needed for digestion and metabolism, and insulin and many other hormones are all made of protein. CHOLESTEROL travels through the bloodstream attached to a lipo- (fat-carrying) protein. A connective tissue made from protein forms the matrix of bones; chromoproteins are a combination of protein and pigments that form hemoglobin; keratin, still another type of protein, is used by the body to make hair and nails. Any dietary protein not needed for these and other functions is stored as fat; some may also be converted to glucose, or blood sugar, and burned for energy.

With so many essential functions allotted to protein, you might assume that it is the number-one nutrient in the diet, but this is not the case. In an ideal balanced diet, only 10 to 12 percent of daily calories should come from protein. Requirements for protein vary according to age, weight, and state of health; on average, a normal adult needs 0.36g of protein per pound of body weight. Thus, a person weighing 140 pounds requires 50g, or slightly less than 2 ounces, of protein per day.

AMINO ACIDS

Proteins are exceedingly complex and diverse structures built of amino acids

---

BENEFITS
- *Used to manufacture and repair all body cells.*
- *Necessary to make antibodies, enzymes, and hormones.*
- *When needed, protein is converted to glucose for energy.*

DRAWBACKS
- *Protein-rich meats and other animal products are often high in fat and cholesterol.*
- *Excessive intake strains the kidneys and liver.*
- *Excessive protein and amino acid supplements increase the excretion of calcium and other minerals.*

---

that are linked together into long chains by peptide bonds. There are many thousands of different proteins, but they all have a backbone of carbon atoms interlaced with nitrogen atoms. Various groupings of atoms can be attached to this backbone.

Human beings need 20 different amino acids; 11 of these can be made in the body, but the other 9, referred to as essential amino acids, must come from the diet. Just as the various letters in the alphabet are joined to make words, so too are amino acids arranged in an almost infinite number of different ways to form the more than 50,000 different proteins in the body. Proteins are made up of hundreds of amino acids. DNA (deoxyribonucleic

acid), the genetic material that is found in the nucleus of each body cell, provides the blueprint for how amino acids are arranged to form individual proteins.

DIETARY PROTEIN

The body is constantly building protein from amino acids, some of which are recycled from the body tissue that is being rebuilt. Even so, a certain amount of protein is lost through normal wear and tear and must be replaced from the diet. But to use this protein, the body must first break it down into its individual amino acids and then reassemble them according to its unique genetic code.

With the exception of oils and pure sugar, all foods contain at least some protein, but its quality varies according to the number of amino acids it provides. Animal protein (with the exception of gelatin) provides all nine essential amino acids in the proportions required by the human body; it is often referred to as complete, or high-quality, protein. In contrast, plant protein (with the exception of soy, which is almost as complete as animal food) lacks one or more of the essential proteins. Because not all plant foods lack the same amino acids, however, the body can build a complete protein if these foods are combined in such a way that they complement each other. For example, grains are high in the essential amino acid methionine, but they lack lysine. This essential amino acid is plentiful in dried beans, peanuts, and other legumes, which are deficient in methionine. So by combining a grain food with a legume, you can obtain the complete range of amino acids.

Interestingly, low-meat ethnic diets all have dishes that provide complementary proteins: the refried beans and corn tortillas of Mexico; the rice and dahl (split peas) of India; the tofu, rice, and vegetable combinations in Asian cuisine; and the chickpeas and bulgur wheat in Middle Eastern dishes. Even strict vegetarian diets can supply ample protein by combining complementary grains and legumes. However, if an essential amino acid is missing from the diet, the body breaks down lean tissue to get it. This may be acceptable on a short-term basis, but over time, it leads to muscle wasting.

Moderate cooking makes protein easier to digest because heat breaks down some of the bonds that join amino acids together. Overcooking, however, can cement some amino acids together, making the protein more difficult to digest and to break down into individual amino acids. Al-

cohol, vinegar, lemon juice, and such enzymes as papain in papayas break some peptide bonds, making these substances good meat tenderizers.

In the stomach, long chains of amino acids are broken into shorter chains called polypeptides. Digestion continues in the small intestine, where pancreatic and other enzymes complete the process. The individual amino acids are absorbed into the bloodstream and transported to the liver, where some are used to make lipoproteins and new enzymes. Others are returned to the bloodstream, which carries them to cells.

Because amino acids are not stored as such, those that are not used in a relatively short time are returned to the liver, where the nitrogen is removed and sent on to the kidneys to be excreted as urea. The remaining protein molecules are stored as fat or converted to glucose for energy.

PROTEIN DEFICIENCY

People in affluent industrialized countries generally consume more than enough protein, but deficiencies are relatively common, especially among children, in rural Africa and other un-

derdeveloped areas where the dietary staples are protein-deficient foods, such as yams, cassava, and other starchy foods. Kwashiorkor, the medical term for severe protein deficiency, is marked by poor growth and mental impairment in children, edema, anemia, muscle wasting, decreased immunity, and metabolic abnormalities.

EXCESSIVE PROTEIN

The typical North American diet provides much more protein than the human body actually needs. This does not pose a serious threat for healthy persons, but too much protein adds to the workload of the kidneys and liver. Thus, people with diseases affecting these organs are generally put on a low-protein diet.

On the down side, meat and other high-protein animal foods come with large amounts of saturated fat and cholesterol—substances that promote atherosclerosis, heart disease, and obesity. Even well-trimmed lean beef derives half of its calories from fat.

SUPPLEMENTS

Purified protein and amino acid powders or pills are often promoted as high-energy, muscle-bulking supplements for athletes and bodybuilders, as well as weight-loss aids for dieters. None of these claims is valid; indeed, taking these supplements can have serious health consequences. In the early 1990s at least 20 deaths were traced to contaminated tryptophan supplements, prompting the Canadian government to ban the sale of individual amino acids. Studies have shown that amino acid supplements can upset normal protein synthesis, setting the stage for nutritional imbalances. Some researchers also maintain that taking amino acid supplements increases calcium excretion and may increase the risk of osteoporosis. Excessive intake of dietary protein may also cause the same problem.

PRUNES

BENEFITS
- *A rich source of vitamin A.*
- *High in B vitamins, vitamin E, potassium, and iron.*
- *Help to relieve constipation.*

DRAWBACKS
- *High in calories.*
- *Leave a sticky residue on the teeth that can lead to cavities.*

Although all prunes are plums, not all plums are prunes. Prunes are the dried fruit from a few particular species of plum trees whose fruit has firm flesh and is naturally high in sugar and acidity. These traits allow the fruit to dry without fermenting if the pit is left in.

Like all dried fruits, prunes contain very little water and are a more concentrated source of energy and nutrients than their fresh fruit counterparts. They are also higher in calories and sugar (a half cup of the stewed fruit or five large pitted prunes contain approximately 115 calories), and they leave a sticky residue on the teeth that can cause cavities. On the plus side, prunes are rich in vitamin A; a 4-ounce serving provides about 50 percent of the Recommended Nutrient Intake (RNI) for adults (in the form of beta carotene), as well as 3mg (30 percent of the RNI) of vitamin E, 3mg of iron, and 750mg of potassium. They are also a good source of B vitamins, magnesium, and phosphorus.

Prunes are popular as a remedy for preventing or treating constipation. This effect can be attributed to prunes' high dietary fiber content; they also contain isatin, a natural laxative.

Unlike other types of juice, prune juice retains most of the fruits' nutrients because it is made by pulverizing the dried prunes and then dissolving them in hot water. One cup of prune juice contains between 20 and 30 percent of the adult RNI of iron and about 700mg of potassium. However, it is also very high in calories, about 200 per cup. Because prune juice is naturally high in sugar, it does not need any additional sweeteners. Although prune juice is not as good a source of fiber as whole prunes, it still helps to relieve constipation because it, too, contains isatin.

PUMPKINS

BENEFITS
- *A rich source of beta carotene.*
- *A good low-calorie source of vitamin C and potassium.*
- *High in fiber.*
- *The seeds are a good source of protein, iron, B vitamins, vitamin E, and fiber.*
- *Can be stored for long periods of time.*

To most Canadians, pumpkins (which are a type of winter squash) are a symbol of Halloween and Thanksgiving. In fact, they have more uses than just as traditional jack-o'-lanterns and pie filling—the strong-flavored flesh of pumpkins can be baked or roasted, used in soups or stews, and turned into a filling for ravioli-style pasta.

Pumpkins were an important food throughout the Americas long before Colonial times. They have been cultivated in Central America for at least 9,000 years, and remains of the fruit have been found in the United States in ancient Southwestern cliff dwellings. Pumpkins are now grown around the world, providing edible flesh, seeds, and flowers; the baby fruit can be baked and consumed whole.

Like all orange-pigmented vegetables, pumpkins are rich in beta carotene, the plant form of vitamin A; a half cup of canned or baked pumpkin provides over 450 percent of the adult Recommended Nutrient Intake (RNI). Studies have shown that this ANTIOXIDANT may help prevent some forms of cancer. Pumpkins are also high in vitamin C; a half-cup serving supplies over 20 percent of the RNI, as well as 275mg of potassium. A half cup has only 40 calories and is very low in fat and high in fiber. Because pumpkins absorb water, they lose some nutrients and have fewer calories per ounce when they are boiled. Sugar pumpkins, which are smaller and sweeter than the large deep-orange pumpkins used for jack-o'-lanterns, are the best choice for cooking and baking.

Although the seeds are often thrown away when a jack-o'-lantern is carved, they are a rich source of protein. One ounce of pumpkin seeds provides 7g of protein—almost as much as an equal serving of peanuts—as well as 3mg of iron (20 to 30 percent of the adult RNI). They are high in unsaturated vegetable oil, a source of vitamin E, and rich in B vitamins. When the coverings are consumed too, the seeds are high in fiber. Pumpkin seeds are easy to prepare: scoop out the seeds, wash them and let dry, then bake them on an oiled baking sheet at 250°F (121°C) for an hour. Commercial varieties are often fried and salted.

Because pumpkins have hard shells, like other winter squashes, they are ideal for storing. Pumpkins last about a month in a cool, dry place. They should not be refrigerated or stored at temperatures below 50°F (10°C), which speeds deterioration.

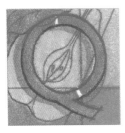

QUINCES

BENEFITS
- *A good source of vitamin C, iron, and potassium.*
- *High in pectin, a soluble fiber.*

DRAWBACKS
- *Often cooked with large amounts of sugar to offset tartness.*
- *Seeds contain a cyanide compound.*

A member of the same rose family as apples and pears, the quince has an acidic tartness that most people find astringent; because of this, the fruit is rarely eaten raw. Cooking, however, cuts the acids, and the fruit takes on a mellow flavor similar to that of a slightly tart apple, with the texture of a pear.

Raw quinces are high in vitamin C; a medium-size fruit provides more than 20mg, or 50 percent of the adult Recommended Nutrient Intake (RNI). Much of this vitamin C is lost, however, when the fruit is cooked. The same-size quince also provides 1mg of iron, which the vitamin C helps the body to absorb, and 305mg of potassium.

The 90 calories in a medium-size quince is comparable to the energy content of apples and pears of the same size. Like these two cousins, quinces are high in pectin, a soluble fiber that helps control blood cholesterol levels and promotes smooth digestive function. Because pectin forms a semisolid gel when cooked, quinces are ideal for making jams and jellies.

Quinces may be round or somewhat pear-shaped. Look for fruit that is firm, with pale yellow skin covered with fuzz; reject any that are small, irregularly shaped, or bruised. The fuzz rubs off easily after the fruit is washed.

Poaching and baking are the most nutritious methods of preparing the fruit. Don't be misled by the tartness of raw quince and add too much sugar. The fruit becomes sweeter as it cooks, so wait until it's done to add a sweetener—you may find you don't need it. Cooking also changes the color of the flesh from pale yellow to pink or red.

Warning: Always remove the quince seeds before cooking. As with apples, apricots, and similar fruits, the seeds contain amygdalin, a compound that turns into hydrogen cyanide in the stomach. Eating a large amount of seeds can result in cyanide poisoning.

QUINOA

BENEFITS
- *An excellent source of iron, magnesium, potassium, phosphorus, zinc, and other minerals.*
- *A good source of B-complex vitamins.*
- *High in protein.*

DRAWBACKS
- *Not widely available and more expensive than most grains.*

Although it is often classified as a grain, quinoa is actually a member of the same plant family as spinach, whereas true grains come from grasses. While the green leafy quinoa (pronounced ki-NOH-wah) tops are edible, it's the seeds that are served most frequently.

For more than 5,000 years, quinoa has been the staple food of the Incas and other native peoples of the Andes, where it is one of the few crops that grows well in the dry mountainous climate and poor soil. It is relatively new

A BITTER COATING

Quinoa seeds taken directly from the plant are inedible because they are coated with a bitter oil containing compounds called saponins. After the seeds are harvested, they are soaked in an alkaline solution to remove the coating. Plant scientists theorize that saponins evolved to protect the seeds from the sun's strong ultraviolet rays at the high altitudes in which the plant grows; the bitter taste also repels birds and bugs.

in North America, however, and in many areas it is still considered an exotic luxury food that is more expensive than most grain products.

The tiny quinoa seeds are packed with important nutrients; a 1-cup serving (made from ¼ cup of dry quinoa) provides about 5mg of iron, more than any unfortified grain product. One cup also contributes large amounts of several other essential minerals, including 100mg of magnesium, 200mg of phosphorus, 370mg of potassium, and 1.5mg of zinc, as well as numerous B vitamins, especially B_6, folate, niacin, and thiamine.

Most of the 160 calories in 1 cup of cooked quinoa come from complex carbohydrates. However, it also provides 7g of protein, which is of a higher quality than similar products because it provides lysine, an amino acid missing in corn, wheat, and other grains.

A VERSATILE FOOD
Quinoa cooks quickly into a fluffy, delicately flavored grainlike dish that lends itself to many uses. It can be served as a substitute for rice, potatoes, and other starchy foods; combined with vegetables, poultry, or seafood to make a pilaf; and added to soups and stews.

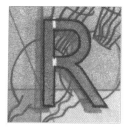

RADISHES

BENEFITS

- *A useful source of vitamin C.*
- *Low in calories and high in fiber.*

DRAWBACKS

- *Can produce gas in some people.*
- *Salicylate content may provoke an allergic reaction in people sensitive to aspirin.*

A member of the cruciferous family, the radish is closely related to cabbage, kale, turnips, and cauliflower. While not especially high in most essential nutrients, radishes are low in calories, making them ideal for snacking and as a spicy addition to salads, soups, and vegetable side dishes.

A useful source of vitamin C, radishes also contain small amounts of iron, potassium, and folate. Four medium-size raw radishes provide 4mg of vitamin C, or 10 percent of the Recommended Nutrient Intake (RNI), and they yield only 5 calories. They also supply sulfurous compounds that may protect against cancer.

Like other cruciferous vegetables, radishes can cause bloating and gas in some people. Also, radishes contain salicylates—compounds similar to the active ingredient in aspirin; many people sensitive to aspirin may suffer an allergic reaction to radishes.

The peak season for radishes spans from April to July, but most varieties are available year-round. Summer radishes have a more intense peppery flavor than those cultivated during spring or fall. Although the bright red globe variety is the best-known in North America, other types include black radishes, daikons, and white icicles.

When selecting red globe radishes, avoid the larger ones if possible, as they may be pithy. A bright color indicates freshness. If there are leaves on the stems, make sure they are green and crisp. Regardless of which variety you are buying, the vegetables should feel solid and have an unblemished surface.

Unless the radishes are going to be served the same day, you should remove any leaves and tops; the radishes will stay fresh longer without the tops. If they are not already packaged, store radishes in plastic bags.

RASPBERRIES

BENEFITS

- *A rich source of vitamin C.*
- *Contain useful amounts of folate, iron, and potassium.*
- *Provide bioflavonoids, which may protect against cancer.*
- *High in fiber.*

DRAWBACKS

- *Contain a natural salicylate, which can cause an allergic reaction in aspirin-sensitive people.*
- *Contain oxalic acid, which can aggravate kidney and bladder stones in susceptible persons.*

There is no sweeter surprise on a summer day than to stumble across a wild raspberry patch. Raspberries—both wild and cultivated—are low in calories and a rich source of vitamin C.

A half-cup serving of raspberries contains 30 calories and 15mg of vitamin C (40 percent of the Recommended Nutrient Intake, or RNI). It also provides 3mcg (micrograms) of folate, 125mg of potassium, and some iron. The vitamin C content increases the iron's absorption, although this may be offset by the oxalic acid in raspberries, which binds with this mineral.

The seeds in raspberries provide an insoluble fiber that helps prevent constipation. The fruit is also high in pectin, a soluble fiber that helps control blood cholesterol levels. In addition, raspberries contain ellagic acid and other bioflavonoids, ANTIOXIDANT plant pigments that may help prevent some types of cancer. Cooking does not destroy ellagic acid, so even raspberry jam may be beneficial.

Raspberries spoil faster than most berries do because of their delicate structure and hollow core. Once picked, they should be eaten as soon as possible. Freezing, however, will preserve them for up to a year.

Cultivated raspberries can be found year-round in gourmet and specialty stores, and when they are in season, at many supermarkets. Before buying raspberries, check that all of them, not just the ones on top, are in good condition; even then, they mold quickly and should be used within 24 hours.

Berries often produce allergic reactions, and raspberries are no exception. Those who are sensitive to aspirin may also react to raspberries, which contain a natural salicylate, similar to the major ingredient in aspirin. Oxalic acid can precipitate kidney and bladder stones in susceptible people; however, it would take a very large amount of raspberries to create problems.

RESTAURANTS AND EATING OUT

*Restaurant meals can be heavy on calories and light
on important nutrients. Plan ahead to avoid nutrition traps,
and patronize restaurants that offer healthy choices.*

For a growing number of Canadians, eating out is no longer just an occasional treat. According to a 1992 government survey, Canadians spent an average of $5,686 per household on meals away from home (this includes restaurants, school cafeterias, and other such establishments).

When dining in a restaurant, people who are following special diets for weight loss or other health needs have to pay attention to the language of menus to bypass nutritional pitfalls—such as excessive calories, fat, and sodium; too few vitamins and minerals; and insufficient fiber. These traps can be avoided by following the guidelines in What to Order for Healthy Eating (facing page). Thanks to consumers' insistence and the growing understanding of nutrition, it's becoming easier to order healthful meals at all types of establishments. Many restaurants now list low-fat dishes and "healthy choices" in a special section of the menu.

The restaurant's staff should be prepared to answer questions about how the food is prepared and to make simple adjustments, such as leaving off sauces and dressings. Restaurants that prepare food to order often cater to special requests, such as dry-broiling fish rather than sautéing it in butter.

DRINKING WITH MEALS

Many people mark special occasions with a restaurant dinner and a celebratory drink or bottle of wine. Although low to moderate ALCOHOL intake (two drinks a day for men and one for women) reduces the risk of a heart attack, excessive drinking leads to serious health problems. It's a good idea, therefore, to quench your thirst with a glass of water before the alcohol and to drink water liberally during the meal. This rehydrates tissues dried out by alcohol and also reduces the temptation to overindulge.

AVOIDING DIET TRAPS

It makes sense to choose a restaurant whose style of food fits the diet that you're following. It's easier, for instance, to order a low-fat meal in a Japanese restaurant than it is in a steak house. The same Japanese meal, however, may supply two to three times the amount of salt that is normally found in Western-style dishes, making it an unwise choice for someone on a low-salt diet.

For many diners, especially when they're hungry, a complimentary basket of breads may be an irresistible temptation. Bread itself contains little fat and, depending on the type, can be a good source of fiber. However, a thick spread of butter or margarine can increase the fat and calories dramatically. Eat the bread plain or ask for a fruit spread instead of butter or margarine. Another good habit is to read the menu as soon as you sit down and order your food right away, thus limiting the time exposed to tempting bread or other fattening appetizers while waiting for your entrée. Or call ahead to ask about the day's specials so you can decide on your entrée in advance; you'll be less tempted to overindulge if you've already made up your mind about what you want.

To avoid overeating, pass up the fixed-price menu and select two or three items from the à la carte menu. Begin with a filling, low-calorie first course—for example, salad, broth-based soup, or shrimp with cocktail

---

BENEFITS

- *Convenient, especially when you are away from home.*
- *Provide a relaxing relief from routine kitchen tasks.*
- *Offer opportunities to sample exotic cuisines.*

DRAWBACKS

- *Expensive, if they take the place of home cooking.*
- *Many dishes are high in calories, fat, and sodium.*
- *May not be appropriate for people on special diets.*

sauce. Many restaurants serve large portions. Don't feel compelled to clean your plate; instead, take the leftovers home. There's no need to pass up dessert, but if you select a high-fat item, share it with your companions.

If you are on a restricted diet, call ahead and ask that a special dish be prepared for you. Most restaurants will accommodate such requests, especially if they have advance notice.

SALAD BARS

Many restaurants have SALAD BARS, which make choices easier for nutrition- and calorie-conscious consumers. Lettuce, spinach, tomatoes, and other fresh vegetables are high in fiber and vitamins and low in calories. It's all too easy, however, to undermine your dietary efforts by overloading the meal with high-calorie toppings and salad dressings, or selecting deli-style potato salad, macaroni salad, and coleslaw, which are made with large quantities of commercial mayonnaise.

FOOD-BORNE ILLNESS

Despite strict laws governing the way food is handled in restaurants, there are still health risks associated with eating out. Managers may follow the letter of the law with regard to cleanliness, but they—like their patrons—are at the mercy of employees who may not always maintain the required standards for hygiene and food handling. You can get a good idea of a restaurant's attention to good hygiene from the general appearance of the dining area. (In some restaurants the kitchen is visible to diners, although it will be partitioned off from the dining area, as required by law.) The staff should appear neatly groomed in clean uniforms and with hair tied back or covered. Soiled table linens, smeared glasses, stale odors, and chipped or discolored plates and utensils are all signs telling the customer to seek out another restaurant.

WHAT TO ORDER FOR HEALTHY EATING

Dining out does not have to be at the expense of balance, moderation, and variety—the tenets of good nutrition. The following suggestions are healthy, tasty alternatives to fatty, unhealthful meals in several popular types of restaurants.

ORDER	INSTEAD OF
NORTH AMERICAN FOOD	
Broth-based soup	Cream soup
An entrée of grilled, broiled, or flame-cooked meat, fish, or poultry	Breaded or batter-dipped meat, fish, or poultry
Sandwiches on whole-wheat or rye bread or a pita	Sandwiches on croissants or biscuits
Baked potato with herbs or margarine	Home-fried or deep-fried potatoes; sour cream or butter
Steamed or baked vegetables	Sautéed or deep-fried vegetables; cream sauces
Salads from the salad bar	Salads made with mayonnaise (coleslaw, pasta, potato, or tuna)
Fresh fruit or frozen yogurt	Pies, cakes, ice cream, or pastries
CHINESE	
Hot and sour soup	Egg rolls
Wonton soup	Fried wontons
Beef with broccoli	Sweet and sour pork or shrimp
Chicken, scallops, or shrimp with vegetables	Peking duck
Steamed rice	Fried rice
ITALIAN	
Minestrone soup	Antipasto platter
Dry breadsticks	Buttered garlic bread
Chicken or fish	Sausage dishes
Pasta with red sauce or clam sauce	Pasta with creamy white or butter sauce
Oil and vinegar dressing	Creamy Italian dressing
Espresso	Cappuccino
Italian ice	Cream-based desserts or pastries
MEXICAN	
Black bean soup	Guacamole dip with taco chips
Burritos, soft tacos, enchiladas, tamales	Tacos, taco salad, tostadas, chili relleños, quesadillas
Soft, plain tortillas	Crispy fried tortillas
Salsa	Sour cream and cheese

Never hesitate to send a dish back if it is undercooked or stale, or if you suspect that it may not have been kept in hygienic conditions. Mistakes can happen in even the best-run establishments, and most restaurant proprietors will be grateful if you bring potential problems to their attention.

RHUBARB

BENEFITS
- *High in vitamin C and potassium.*

DRAWBACKS
- *Usually prepared with substantial amounts of sugar or other sweeteners.*
- *Contains oxalic acid, which inhibits calcium and iron absorption.*
- *Leaves are highly poisonous.*

Although rhubarb is generally regarded as a fruit, botanically it is a vegetable. It is available in frozen and canned forms, but most people prefer to cook the fresh stalks themselves. One cup of fresh diced rhubarb yields a mere 26 calories and provides 10mg of vitamin C (25 percent of the adult Recommended Nutrient Intake, or RNI), as well as 350mg of potassium. This same serving size also contains more than 100mg of calcium; however, rhubarb is not considered a good source of this mineral, since it also contains oxalic acid, which not only blocks the absorption of its calcium but also that from any other dietary sources. Because it has a high oxalic acid content, large amounts of rhubarb should be avoided by anyone with a tendency to develop oxalate-containing kidney stones or bladder stones.

Only the rhubarb stalks are eaten—the leaves are highly poisonous. Because raw rhubarb stalks are stringy in texture and tart in flavor, most people will consume them only when cooked with large amounts of sugar or honey, thus inflating the calorie count.

One cup of cooked sweetened rhubarb yields 280 calories. To avoid extra calories, try cooking the stalks with sweet fruits, such as strawberries or apples.

A favorite springtime pie filling, rhubarb can also be made into preserves, or it can be stewed to make a compote or sauces to complement poultry, other meat dishes, and desserts.

When cooked and sweetened, rhubarb will turn brownish in color. It should not be prepared in aluminum or cast iron pots, which will interact with the acid in the vegetable and darken both the pot and the rhubarb.

RICE

BENEFITS
- *Enriched varieties provide B vitamins and iron.*
- *Makes a complete protein when combined with beans and other legumes.*
- *Gluten-free and suitable for people with celiac disease.*
- *Easy to digest and useful in restoring bowel function after a bout of diarrhea.*
- *Rarely, if ever, causes food allergies.*

DRAWBACKS
- *Diets high in white rice may be deficient in thiamine.*
- *Brown rice is more nutritious but takes longer to cook than white rice.*
- *A substance in brown rice can inhibit absorption of iron and calcium.*

For thousands of years, rice has been the staple food for more than half the world's population. In some Asian countries per capita consumption exceeds 300 pounds a year, and survival still depends on the rice crop. In contrast, the average Canadian eats only about 27 pounds of rice a year, which includes all types of rice, as well as breakfast cereals.

Like barley and oats, rice grows in a protective husk that has to be removed if the grain is to be used as food. (Wheat, rye, and corn, by contrast, are bare seeds that require less processing.) Many nutrients are lost with the bran and germ that are removed in milling to make white rice. Brown rice—intact kernels that retain their bran layers—is somewhat more nutritious than white rice, but it also contains phytic acid, a substance that interferes with the absorption of iron and calcium.

Although not grown in Canada, most of the white rice that is grown and processed in the United States is fortified with iron, niacin, and thiamine, which are applied in a solution to the outside of the grain, coated with a protein powder, and dried. Rinsing the grain before cooking washes away these important nutrients. Rice should be cooked in just twice its volume of water, which will be completely absorbed by the grain and will preserve the nutritional content.

Converted rice is processed by a 2,000-year-old method; this involves parboiling the whole grain, which makes milling easier by loosening the husk. Conversion improves the nutritional quality of the grain by causing the B vitamins in the bran and germ to permeate the endosperm. It also gelatinizes the fat- and nutrient-bearing aleurone layer, which then adheres to the grain instead of being lost with the bran. Thanks to this technique, the thiamine deficiency known as beriberi was never a serious threat to people in India and Pakistan, although it ravaged Asian people who subsisted on unconverted white rice. Instant rice should

THE LONG AND THE SHORT OF IT.
Varieties of rice include: (left row, from top) instant long-grain white, long-grain brown, instant basmati, and risotto; (middle row, from top) long-grain white, instant long-grain brown, and glutinous brown; (right row, from top) long-grain white, wild, soft pudding, brown basmati, and basmati.

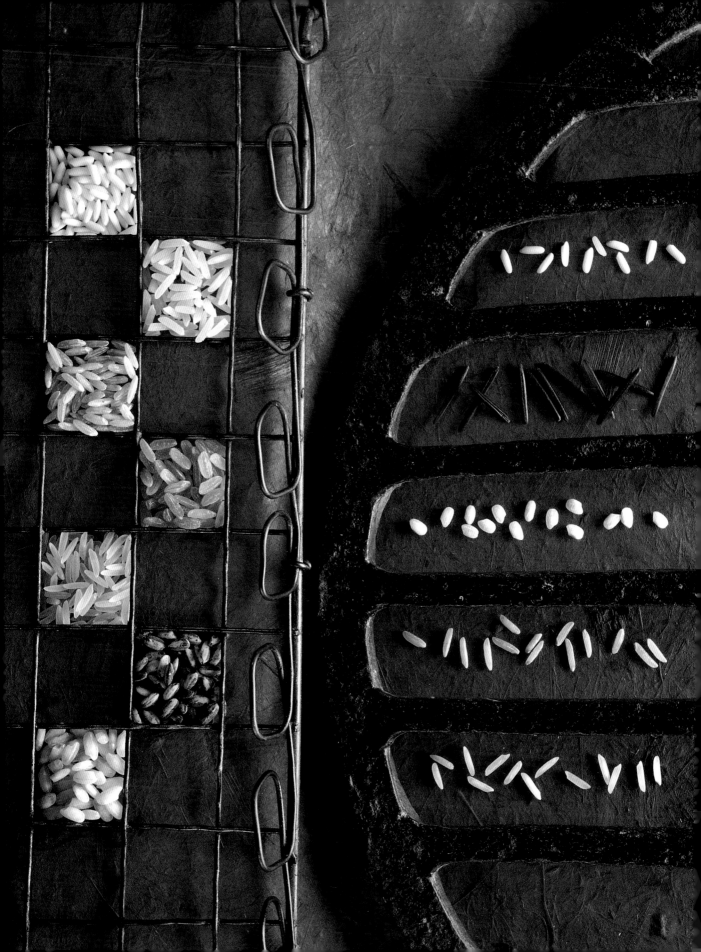

not be confused with converted rice, which takes at least as long to cook as other types. Much of the rice sold in Canada is also polished in special machines to make it shiny. An extra sheen is achieved by coating the grains with talc and glucose. This is a cosmetic process with no nutritional impact.

NUTRITIONAL VALUE

Ninety percent of the calories in rice come from carbohydrates. A half cup of cooked rice constitutes one of the 5 to 12 daily servings of carbohydrates recommended in the Food Guide Rainbow (see p.23). A half cup of white rice contains about 100 calories, while brown rice may have 105 to 110. Brown rice is significantly higher in fiber, with 1.6g per half cup compared to 0.03g in the same volume of white rice.

The protein content of rice, ranging from 2.0 to 2.5mg per half cup, is less than that of other cereals, but the amino acid balance is superior to that of other grains. Processed rice contains only a trace of fat and no sodium.

Macrobiotic regimens were FAD DIETS in the 1960s; the most restrictive seventh level of the diets provides little else but brown rice. It fell out of favor when people became aware of the serious nutritional deficiencies created when some individuals adopted this strict level. Like other carbohydrates, rice must be counterbalanced with foods from the other compartments of the Food Guide Rainbow to provide a complete range of vitamins, minerals, and protein.

HEALTH BENEFITS

Rice has a binding effect in diarrhea, and as such, is part of the BRAT (for banana, rice, applesauce, and toast) diet. It helps restore normal bowel function and provides needed energy for someone recovering from diarrhea. Rice pudding made with low-fat milk and flavored with cinnamon is a soothing, easy-to-digest dish for convalescents.

Several studies have shown that rice bran helps to reduce cholesterol and may reduce the risk of bowel cancer. Some studies also show that rice helps regulate glucose metabolism in people with diabetes. As a complex carbohydrate, it provides a slow, steady supply of glucose, and not the rapid rise that occurs after eating sugars.

Along with lamb and a few other foods, rice rarely if ever provokes an allergic reaction. This quality makes rice ideal as the basis of the strict elimination diet that is sometimes used to identify food allergens.

A VERSATILE STAPLE

Rice is a true staple in menu planning. Risotto, made with fat-free broth and vegetables, and pilaf, based on fat-free broth, chopped nuts, and dried fruits, are economical, nutritious, low-fat entrées. Rice is an ingredient of hot and cold breakfast cereals, an excellent base for salads, and a natural companion to vegetables, fish, meats, and cheese. Rice bran also adds bulk to baked goods.

RICE VARIETIES

Rice is classified by size and shape (long, medium, and short grain). Long-grain rice remains dry and separate when cooked; short-grain rice, which is wetter and stickier, is more often used in Asian and Caribbean cooking.

Arborio rice is a creamy-textured, medium-grain Italian rice used in making risotto because it remains firm at the center through long cooking.

Basmati is an aromatic rice native to Pakistan and India. When cooked, the grain swells only lengthwise. Basmati grains stay dry and separate and are especially suitable for pilafs.

Jasmine is an aromatic rice with origins in Thailand. It has a soft, moist texture and grains that cling together.

Wild rice, a very distant relative of common rice, is a grass native to the lakes and marshes of the Great Lakes region. Once gathered by hand in the wild by Chippewa Indians, wild rice is now cultivated commercially and harvested by machine. Wild rice contains more protein than common rice does and is richer in lysine, the amino acid lacking in most grains.

DID YOU KNOW?

- We commemorate an ancient Asian fertility symbol when we shower bridal couples with rice.

- Wild rice grows in marshlands and waterways from Manitoba to the Atlantic Ocean. It is one of the few wild plant foods harvested and marketed in Canada.

- Rice is an important component of many commercially produced baby foods, because it is easy to digest and hypoallergenic.

- According to legend, rice was accidentally introduced to the Americas when a storm-stricken ship docked in Charleston, South Carolina, and the captain gave some seeds to a local planter.

- The outer, most nutritious parts of the rice kernel are removed and fed to livestock when rice is milled.

- Broken grains of rice are used for brewing beer.

SALAD BARS—THE MANY PROS AND CONS

*Although typical salad bar offerings are perceived
as healthy alternatives to fast foods,
a number of them are loaded with fat and salt.*

Once considered a trendy fad in family restaurants, the salad bar is now as ubiquitous as fast-food eateries. Even chic high-priced restaurants have set up salad bars; they're also found in fast-food establishments, delicatessens, and a variety of institutional settings. Many salad bars provide complete meals, with everything from soups and relishes, raw and cooked vegetables and fruits, to hot and cold entrées, and even desserts.

There are advantages to such a set-up. It allows diners to put together their own meals without having to wait, and it enables restaurants to cut staffing costs. But there are also some drawbacks, especially for those watching their fat intake and weight. Although most people regard salads as low-calorie dishes that can be eaten with impunity, the fact is, many salad bar meals have more fat and calories than a hamburger and French fries. It's all a matter of what you pick and which dressings and toppings you use.

PRACTICING RESTRAINT

Salad bar devotees say there's an art to creating a healthful meal from the 50 or more selections at a typical setup. Many people make the mistake of going to a salad bar when they're hungry, and then starting at one end and dishing up whatever looks appealing until their plate or takeout container is overflowing. A better approach is to survey the offerings and plan your

---

BENEFITS

- *Many offer a wide choice of greens, fresh vegetables, and fruits.*
- *Consumers can create their own salad or entrée, usually for less than it costs to order from the restaurant's regular menu.*

DRAWBACKS

- *Many choices are high in fat and sodium.*
- *The temptation to sample many offerings can result in overeating.*
- *Foods may be exposed to flies and other disease-carrying pests.*
- *There's a risk of food poisoning from items allowed to stand at room temperature for more than an hour or two.*

---

meal. If you're creating a salad to complement a restaurant meal, concentrate on a modest beginning—perhaps some raw vegetables or an assortment of greens with a low-calorie dressing. Remember, your main dish will probably be served with vegetables or other side dishes, so you don't need to fill up before it arrives.

Even if you're making an entire meal from the salad bar, you should still survey the choices and plan your menu before you start loading your plate. Decide on a single main dish—for example, a helping of lasagna, chili, broiled fish, or sliced turkey (all common salad bar offerings). Then

plan what you want to accompany it: perhaps a green salad or slice of melon as a first course; steamed or raw vegetables, a baked potato, or a serving of rice as side dishes; and sorbet or fresh fruit for dessert. Only after you've planned your meal should you start putting food on your plate. Begin with small helpings; many salad bars allow repeat trips, so you can always go back for more if you're still hungry.

You should use the same approach if you're assembling a take-out meal. Even though you won't be able to go back for seconds, you should still limit yourself to those selections that will form a balanced meal. Emphasize complex carbohydrates and add plenty of raw or lightly cooked vegetables, fresh fruit, and a modest serving of lean meat, poultry, seafood, or other high-protein selection.

TOPPINGS AND DRESSINGS

A 100-calorie plate of greens, vegetables, and, perhaps, fruits can be transformed into an 880-calorie meal (with very little added nutrition but extra calories and fat) by topping it with an ounce of croutons (120 calories), 2 tablespoons of blue cheese (180 calories), an ounce of sunflower seeds (160 calories), and ¼ cup of regular Italian dressing (320 calories). Instead, you can achieve a similar taste by adding 1 tablespoon of Parmesan cheese (23 calories), 2 tablespoons of sliced mushrooms (2 calories), 2 tablespoons of raw onions (7 calories), and 2 table-spoons of low-calorie Italian dressing (14 calories), for only 146 calories. Of course, many salad bar offerings have already been mixed, often with high-fat ingredients and dressings. Reject vegetables and other foods surrounded by oil, butter, or other fat. The high sheen on steamed or sautéed vegetables usually comes from oil, which is added to keep the foods from looking dry and withered. It's also a good bet that too much mayonnaise has been used to make egg, tuna, chicken, and seafood salads; avoid these items unless they're labeled as having been made with a low-fat dressing.

SALAD BAR SAFETY

In the past a number of severe asthma attacks were traced to salad bar foods sprayed with sulfites to preserve their color and freshness. Sulfites are no longer used for this purpose, but people with severe food allergies, celiac disease, and other food sensitivities still need to approach salad bars and cafeteria-type setups with caution; their offerings may be made with hidden offending ingredients, such as flour, wheat, and cornstarch.

Each year millions of North Americans suffer bouts of food poisoning, and many of these are linked to open salad bars. Fortunately, most such incidents are short-lived, but some people—the very young, the elderly, and anyone with a chronic debilitating disease or lowered immunity—can suffer more serious consequences and may be well-advised to forgo salad bars or to select products in sealed containers.

When inspecting a salad bar, look for clues, such as withered greens and dried-out pasta, that might indicate if the food has been standing too long. Does the bar's surface feel cold (a sign that it's refrigerated or filled with ice)? Are there flies or evidence of other insects? If in doubt, go elsewhere or order freshly prepared food.

WISE SALAD BAR CHOICES

Most salad bars offer a few low-calorie choices and a wide range of tempting, high-fat alternatives. Use the following guide to create a healthful, interesting meal that's not overweighted with high-fat foods.

LOW-CALORIE OPTION	CALORIES	HIGH-CALORIE ALTERNATIVE	CALORIES
CONDIMENTS/TOPPINGS (2 tbsp)			
Alfalfa sprouts	2	Sunflower seeds	160
Anchovies (3)*	20	Bacon bits*	55
Chopped egg	25	Croutons* (1 oz)	120
Dill pickles (1 medium)*	5	Green olives* (8)	30
Parmesan cheese*	45	Blue cheese*	180
Raw chopped onion	7	Shredded Cheddar cheese*	55
DRESSINGS (1 tbsp)			
Garlic yogurt*	25	Cheese garlic*	90
Low-fat blue cheese*	11	Regular blue cheese*	75
Low-fat French*	22	Regular French*	65
Low-fat herb*	20	Caesar*	75
Low-fat Italian*	7	Regular Italian*	80
Low-fat vinaigrette*	8	Classic vinaigrette*	45
Nonfat mayonnaise*	20	Regular mayonnaise*	100
FRUITS, DESSERTS			
Applesauce (½ cup)	75	Apple pie	280
Chocolate chip cookie	50	Chocolate pudding (½ cup)	175
Fruit ice (½ cup)	80	Strawberry ice cream	270
SALADS (½ CUP)			
Carrot-raisin	45	Pasta (with mayonnaise)*	165
Fresh fruit	30	Waldorf (fruit, nut)	185
Mixed greens	10	Greek (with olives)*	95
Pickled beets	70	Potato (with mayonnaise)*	180
Red cabbage	30	Coleslaw	125
Tofu with chopped peppers	60	Lentil (with oil)*	140
Tomato-cucumber	25	Chickpeas (with oil)	160
Water-packed tuna*	120	Oil-packed tuna*	190
SOUPS (1 CUP)			
Beef barley*	60	Cream of mushroom*	315
Chicken noodle*	75	Cream of chicken*	200
Vegetable*	85	Split pea with ham*	250
SPECIALTY ITEMS			
Baked potato with herbs	140	Baked potato with cheese	520
Calamari (marinated)	140	Calamari (deep fried)	250
Fish fillet (baked)	90	Fish (breaded, deep fried)	200
Sushi (rice, vegetable)	40	Fried Chinese dumpling	150

Note: Calorie values vary from place to place; those quoted here are an average.

* High in sodium unless labeled low-salt.

STRESS: STRATEGIES FOR COPING

Prolonged stress, whether psychological or physical, plays havoc with digestion and nutritional needs. Certain foods can provide the extra energy or comfort needed to get through a stressful period.

When people talk about stress, they are usually referring to tension or emotional distress. Medically, however, stress is defined as any condition or situation that places undue strain on the body. The sources can be a physical illness or injury, as well as numerous psychological factors—including fear, feelings of anger or frustration, and even unusual happiness. What constitutes almost unbearable stress to one person may be the spice of life to someone else. In either case, a stressor (a stimulus that causes stress) can trigger the body's automatic stress-response system. This sets the stage for decreased immune resistance and increased vulnerability to illnesses, ranging from the common cold to heart attacks and cancer.

While physical stress is often episodic, emotional stress is part of daily life. This is not a modern phenomenon. Our early ancestors experienced much more stress than we do—from the constant quest for food to dangers from hostile neighbors and wild animals. While we don't usually encounter such situations, our bodies will still respond to any stress much as they would have in prehistoric times. This stress-coping mechanism, called the fight-or-flight response, floods the body with adrenaline and other hormones that raise blood pressure, speed up the heartbeat, tense muscles, and put other systems on alert. Metabolism quickens to provide extra energy; digestion stops as blood is diverted from the intestines to the muscles.

NUTRITIONAL NEEDS

Diet plays a critical role in helping the body deal with stress. In fact, stress quickly exhausts the body's supply of glucose, its major fuel. Once this happens, the body starts to break down the protein in muscles, a quicker source of energy than body fat. Consequently, extra CARBOHYDRATES, both sugars and starches, are required to provide fast energy. In addition, extra dietary PROTEIN, preferably from lean meat, fish, low-fat milk, and egg whites, is needed to help prevent muscle wasting. (Vegetarians can get protein from tofu and combinations of grains and lentils, dried beans and peas, and other legumes.) Unfortunately, prolonged stress can diminish

---

ARE YOU STRESSED?

Because stress can cause many different symptoms, both physical and mental, it's often difficult to determine their true source. A doctor may order medical tests, even if he suspects that stress is the real problem. The following are common manifestations of stress:

Physical symptoms
• Palpitations, shortness of breath, chest pain, and other signs of heart disease (which must be ruled out).
• High blood pressure.
• Unusual rapid breathing, dizziness, or light-headedness.
• Tingling sensations in the hands and/or feet.
• Chronic or recurring backache and neck pain.
• Frequent headaches.
• Diarrhea or constipation.
• Heartburn and other types of digestive problems.

• An increased vulnerability to colds and other illnesses.

Psychological symptoms
• Unexplained irritability or feelings of sadness.
• Difficulty in concentrating and in making decisions.
• Sleep problems.
• Chronic fatigue, even after adequate rest.
• Prolonged anxiety.
• Changes in appetite and an increased reliance on alcohol, nicotine, or other drugs.
• Difficulty coping with what are normally minor setbacks.
• Needless worrying over even trivial problems.
• Decreased enjoyment of pleasurable activities and events.
• A diminished interest in sex.
• An increased likelihood of being in accidents.

appetite, further compounding the problem of muscle loss.

A balanced diet that provides ample fruits, vegetables, and whole-grain products compensates for any nutrients that were lost because of stress and meets the body's increased need for vitamins A and C and for thiamine, riboflavin, and other B vitamins. Stress also prompts the kidneys to increase the secretion of important minerals, in particular calcium, zinc, and magnesium. Contrary to advertising claims, taking high doses of so-called antistress vitamins will not calm jittery nerves.

When under stress, some people are always hungry and binge on food; others have to force themselves to eat. Because stress interferes with digestion, it's better to eat four to six small meals spaced throughout the day instead of the traditional three large ones. A varied diet of mostly complex carbohydrates and protein provides essential energy and nutrients and is easier to digest than a high-fat one.

COMFORT FOODS

Almost everyone has a favorite food that provides comfort during stressful times; the choices vary from one person to the next. For some people, it's a food that harks back to childhood, such as milk. Others crave chocolate or sweets, which increase the production of serotonin, a brain chemical that has a calming effect. Soups are also favorite choices, as are bland, easy-to-digest foods like rice pudding, custards, yogurt, and omelets. Experiment and go with whatever works best for you.

BETTER OFF WITHOUT

Because stress can play havoc with normal digestion, foods that normally are well tolerated may trigger indigestion and heartburn. Fatty foods, which are difficult to digest at any time, should be avoided. Many people also find that hot or spicy foods cause problems during times of stress.

Avoid ALCOHOL, caffeine drinks, and cigarettes. These substances are stimulants that can add to jittery feelings. Instead, try a herbal tea, low-fat milk, fruit juice, or a noncaffeinated soft drink.

COMFORT FOODS. *Quietly relaxing with a cup of herbal tea is a time-honored stress beater. A carbohydrate snack of toast or a similar food helps restore depleted glucose supplies.*

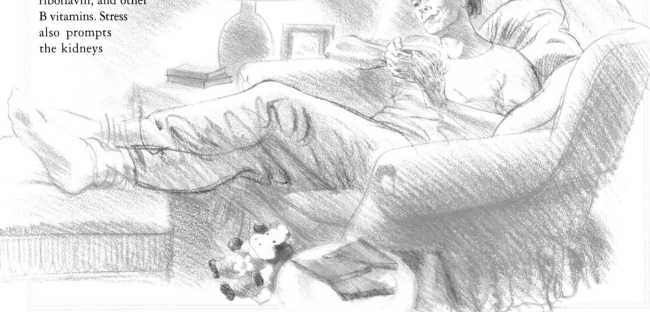

STROKE

EAT PLENTY OF

- *Fresh fruits and vegetables for vitamin C and other antioxidants.*
- *Nuts, seeds, green leafy vegetables, wheat germ, and fortified cereals for vitamin E; these foods plus bananas and other fruits for potassium.*
- *Oily fish for omega-3 fatty acids.*
- *Oat bran, legumes, and fruits for pectin and other soluble fibers.*
- *Onions and garlic, which may help to prevent blood clots.*

CUT DOWN ON

- *Animal and dairy products that are high in saturated fats and cholesterol.*
- *Salt, which may raise blood pressure.*
- *Alcohol use.*

AVOID

- *Smoking.*
- *Excessive weight gain.*

Each year more than 500,000 North Americans suffer strokes, roughly one every minute. In Canada, strokes claim over 14,000 lives annually, making stroke our third leading cause of death (exceeded only by heart attacks and cancer). Approximately 80 percent of all strokes occur when a clot blocks blood flow to a part of the brain. Most of these clots form in an artery that is already narrowed by atherosclerosis, either in the brain itself or, more commonly, in the carotid artery in the neck. The remaining 20 percent are hemorrhagic strokes, in which there is bleeding in the brain, such as from a burst blood vessel or severe head injury. Hemorrhagic strokes, which are more likely to be fatal than those caused by clots, are more common in people with high blood pressure.

The warning signs of a stroke include sudden weakness or numbness of the face, arm, and leg on one side of the body; difficulty speaking or understanding others; dimness or impaired vision in one eye; and unexplained dizziness, unsteadiness, or a sudden fall. Immediate treatment is critical, even if the symptoms disappear, as in the case of a ministroke (transient ischemic attack), a common prelude to a full-blown stroke. Prompt treatment may be lifesaving, and it may also minimize permanent damage, which can include impaired movement, speech, vision, and mental function.

PREVENTIVE MEASURES

The death rate for stroke has been cut to less than half of what it was in 1950, thanks largely to a better understanding of the underlying causes, especially the key risk factors, such as high blood pressure, heart disease, arteriosclerosis, and diabetes. A number of unhealthy lifestyle habits also increase the risk of a stroke; these include smoking, excessive use of ALCOHOL, obesity, and a sedentary lifestyle.

Diet plays an important role in reducing or eliminating these risk factors. In fact, many of the same nutritional recommendations made for people who have heart disease, high blood pressure, and elevated blood CHOLESTEROL levels apply to people at risk for, or who have had, a stroke. A good starting point is to adopt a diet that is low in fats, especially saturated animal fats and tropical (palm and coconut) oils. About 60 percent of calories should come from carbohydrates, with emphasis on such starchy foods as pasta, grains, and legumes, along with five to ten daily servings of fruits and vegetables. These foods are high in the soluble fibers that help control cholesterol levels and reduce the risk of atherosclerosis, which narrows the arteries and sets the stage

REDUCING THE RISKS. *The key to avoiding stroke is a diet low in salt and saturated fat and high in fiber and the omega-3 fatty acids found in some oils and oily fish.*

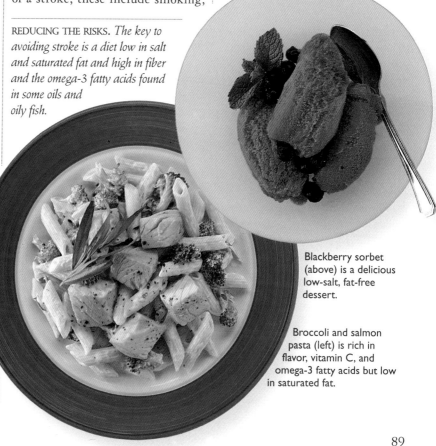

Blackberry sorbet (above) is a delicious low-salt, fat-free dessert.

Broccoli and salmon pasta (left) is rich in flavor, vitamin C, and omega-3 fatty acids but low in saturated fat.

for developing the blood clots that block the flow of blood to the brain.

A number of foods appear to lower the risk of a stroke. Some fish, for example, are rich in omega-3 fatty acids, which help to prevent blood clots by reducing the stickiness of blood platelets. Doctors recommend eating salmon, trout, mackerel, sardines, or other oily cold-water fish two or three times a week. Other good sources of omega-3 fatty acids include wheat germ, walnuts and walnut oil, canola (rapeseed) oil, soybeans, and purslane (a popular salad green in a number of Mediterranean countries).

Garlic and onions appear to decrease the tendency of the blood to clot, and they also boost the body's natural clot-dissolving mechanism. A Chinese mushroom called the tree ear may have similar beneficial effects. This mushroom is available dried in Chinese markets and gourmet shops, and when rehydrated with a little boiling water, it makes a tasty addition to soups, stews, and casseroles. A recent study found that a tablespoon of the soaked mushroom consumed three or four times a week may be as effective in preventing strokes and heart attacks as a daily aspirin—but without the risk of gastrointestinal irritation.

A growing body of scientific evidence shows that vitamin E, too, reduces the tendency to form blood clots. Foods high in this ANTIOXIDANT include nuts, seeds, wheat germ, fortified grain products, and green leafy vegetables. Other antioxidants include vitamin C, which strengthens blood vessel walls and thus may protect against brain hemorrhages; most fruits (especially citrus) and vegetables are good sources. Many of these foods, as well as grains and legumes, are high in potassium, an electrolyte instrumental in maintaining normal blood pressure.

Anyone who has high blood pressure, or a family history of this disease

or of strokes, should limit salt intake; excessive sodium—a main component of salt—increases the body's fluid volume and may raise blood pressure.

Numerous studies link excessive alcohol use, defined as more than two drinks a day for men and one for women, to an increased incidence of stroke; the risk is compounded if the person also smokes. The best approach is to abstain completely from smoking and to use alcohol only in moderation, if at all. Regular exercise not only reduces the risk of a stroke and heart attack by helping control weight and blood cholesterol levels, but it also fosters an enhanced sense of well-being.

SUGAR AND OTHER SWEETENERS

BENEFITS
- *Sugar satisfies an inborn taste for sweets.*
- *Artificial sweeteners satisfy our sweet tooth without adding calories.*

DRAWBACKS
- *Excess sugar may be consumed instead of useful nutrients and lead to obesity.*
- *Sugar fosters the growth of cavity-causing bacteria.*

Refined sugar is a relatively new food in the human diet, becoming widely available only since the 1500s. It didn't take long for this sweetener to become a major commodity, and for tooth decay to reach epidemic proportions.

Sugars have been described as a "standard currency" for living organisms, because all plants and animals store energy chemically as sugar. The sugars adapted for our diet are natural substances produced by photosynthesis in plants. Nutrition experts distinguish two main types of sugar: intrinsic sugar,

which gives an appealing taste to such foods as fruits and sweet vegetables, and extrinsic sugar, which is added to food during preparation or processing or at the time of consumption.

Sugarcane and sugar beets are our main sources of sugar; some liquid sweeteners, such as molasses, are by-products of sugar refining. Manufacturers favor liquid sweeteners made from corn or potatoes because their sweetness and thickness can be regulated. They add a chewy texture to foods, and they prevent moisture loss and extend the shelf life of products.

The main sugar in our diet is sucrose, familiar to us as white sugar. But contrary to popular belief, Canadians on average do not consume too much sugar. In fact, sugar consumption has changed little since the 1920s. The average Canadian consumes about 10 to 15 percent of total calories from added sugars, an amount consistent with generally recommended guidelines. Consumption is highest in younger age groups, contributing about 13 to 15 percent of calories, and declining to approximately 9 percent of calories after age 50.

FOOD VALUE
At 99.9 percent sucrose, white sugar is an extremely pure food. Sucrose is a disaccharide (double sugar) made up of two monosaccharides (single sugars): glucose (known as blood sugar, dextrose, or grape sugar) and fructose (the sugar in fruits and maple sap).

The intrinsic sugars in fruits, vegetables, and starches are bound up with essential vitamins, minerals, fiber, and oils. Extrinsic sugar, however, contains empty calories that can supply energy, but it provides no valuable nutrients, although it satisfies our taste for sweetness and can enhance the flavor of many foods. And while many of the evils blamed on sugar—hyperactivity, acne, high blood pressure, obesity—have

ARTIFICIAL SWEETENERS

Although sugar substitutes are considered safe for adults, children should not use them, because it's difficult for their smaller bodies to eliminate substances that may possibly be harmful.

• **Acesulfame-K** passes through the body unchanged, and is therefore noncaloric. Two hundred times sweeter than sugar, it withstands heat and can be used for baking.

• **Aspartame** contains the same calories, weight for weight, as sugar, but since it is 200 times sweeter, it can provide a teaspoon's worth of sweetness with only one-tenth of a calorie. Aspartame loses its sweetness when cooked or exposed to certain acids. Aspartame is unsafe for people with phenylketonuria (PKU), and it should be avoided by people with epilepsy.

• **Cyclamates** are allowed in Canada, but not in the United States. Studies associating them with an increased risk of bladder cancer led to their removal from the U.S. market. But many researchers, and the Canadian government, believe that these studies were flawed and that the compounds are safer than saccharin.

• **Saccharin.** The body cannot absorb saccharin; instead, it is excreted by the kidneys. Although very high doses have been associated with bladder cancer in rats, saccharin has been in use for so long that most experts consider the risk to be low for adults using normal amounts. In Canada, saccharin is allowed as a tabletop sweetener only.

• **Sucralose** is 600 times sweeter than sugar. Since it is not absorbed by the body, it is calorie-free. It is allowed in Canada both as an additive in beverages and processed foods, and as a tabletop sweetener.

been found to be unrelated or only indirectly linked through overconsumption, it is true that sugar is a major cause of dental disorders and that people who turn to sugary fast foods for a quick energy boost may neglect less convenient but much more nutritious foods.

All forms of sugar provide about the same energy value: 4 calories per gram. In everyday terms, a cup of white sugar contains 770 calories, compared to 820 in a cup of densely packed brown sugar. A tablespoon of white sugar has 45 calories, and an individual serving packet, 25. Although sugar itself is not especially high in calories, many sweet foods, such as chocolates and pastries, are also high in fat, which contains 9 calories per gram.

Confectioners' sugar has about 385 calories in a cup. Although the sugar is pure sucrose, the product is packaged with cornstarch to prevent clumping. Because of this, people with ALLERGIC REACTIONS to corn may suffer adverse reactions from the powdered sugar in frostings and desserts. Raw sugar—the first crystals obtained during the refining process—is not sold in Canada because it is contaminated with soil, plant refuse, and insect droppings and parts. Turbinado sugar, available in health-food stores, is raw sugar that has been purified.

Contrary to the claims of natural-food enthusiasts, neither brown sugar nor honey is more nutritious than white sugar, but consumers who find the taste more appealing can substitute brown for white sugar in any recipe. Brown sugar is made by coating white sugar crystals with molasses. While molasses contains iron and other minerals, the amount in brown sugar is too small to be of nutritional value.

MAPLE SUGAR

Maple sugar and syrup are made by boiling down maple sap—a technique developed by North America's native people long before the arrival of white explorers. Pure maple products are expensive because production is limited. A tablespoon of maple syrup contains 50 calories, and 1 ounce of maple sugar has 100. Pure maple products contain traces of potassium, calcium, and other minerals, but not in amounts sufficient to be of much nutritional value.

DENTAL PROBLEMS

All types of sugar—white table sugar, brown sugar, honey, molasses—encourage the growth of the oral bacteria that are responsible for causing dental caries. And when starchy foods are broken down by the enzymes in saliva, they, too, form cavity-causing sugars. More dangerous than the amount of sugar is the length of time the sugar remains in contact with the teeth. Thus, much of the damage can be prevented by brushing soon after eating a sweet.

Sugar alcohols, such as sorbitol, that are used as sweeteners in commercial products do not cause cavities, but do contribute calories. Xylitol—not available by itself but used in sugar-free products, including gum—seems to protect against tooth decay. Other sugar substitutes were thought to be beneficial only because they are not broken down into acids in the mouth, but studies in laboratory animals show that saccharin, like xylitol, may actually protect against cavities.

A UNIQUE SWEETENER

Artichokes contain cynarin, a unique organic acid that stimulates sweetness receptors in the taste buds. After eating artichokes, some people find that everything—including plain water—tastes sweet for a short time. However, efforts to convert this natural substance into a commercial sugar substitute have not yet been successful.

SUPPLEMENTS—WHO NEEDS THEM?

Nutritionists maintain that vitamin and mineral pills are unnecessary for most people. So why do so many Canadians persist in taking them, often in very high doses?

Millions of Canadians take nutritional supplements, usually without the advice of a doctor. Some take supplements because they fear their diets may be lacking; others believe that if a little of something is good, a lot must be even better. What many people don't know is that a varied diet based on the Food Guide Rainbow (see p.23) provides all the nutrients a healthy person needs. In fact, if someone consumes more nutrients than his body can use or store, the excess is usually excreted in the urine and feces. And when taken in large amounts, some supplements—for example, iron and vitamins A and D—are highly toxic.

Nutritionists stress that the diet is the best source of the necessary vitamins, minerals, fatty acids, amino acids, and fiber, because, as components of food, they come packaged with a host of other chemicals. Some of these substances promote the absorption of a nutrient; others delay it. In any case, the natural form of the food is usually the one best adapted to the human digestive system. In contrast, supplements contain only one form of a nutrient and lack the other chemicals, energy, fiber, and dietary components that provide a proper nutritional balance.

People who depend on vitamin and mineral supplements to compensate for gaps in their daily dietary intake may not understand the principles of sound nutrition. The recommended daily servings in the Food Guide Rainbow are actually based on the desirable average of food consumption over the course of about 2 weeks. The liver, which stores vitamins and minerals, can make up for any occasional dietary lapses by releasing stored nutrients as they are needed. Well-nourished people typically have enough stored vitamins and minerals for at least 3 months of deprivation before they begin to develop symptoms of deficiency diseases.

In the early years of this century, such diseases as pellagra (caused by a lack of niacin) and beriberi (a thiamine deficiency disease) were widespread in some regions and income groups. After these essential B vitamins and other nutrients were added to refined grain products and other common foods, such deficiency diseases all but disappeared except in special situations, such as alcoholism or other diseases that foster malnutrition.

One exception is iron-deficiency ANEMIA, which is relatively common in young women worldwide because of their monthly blood loss through menstruation. Most of these women do not need iron supplements, however; a diet that includes such iron-rich foods as lean meat, poultry, fish, enriched breads and cereals, and legumes can prevent anemia.

USEFUL SUPPLEMENTS

Even though most people do not need supplements, there are a few exceptions. Sometimes doctors advise individuals on low-calorie weight-loss diets to take daily multivitamin supplements that provide no more than 100 percent of the Recommended Nutrient Intakes (RNIs) for any nutrient. Similarly, supplements may be recommended for elderly people, who may have poor appetites or metabolic problems, or for convalescents, who

---

BENEFITS
- *May hasten recovery in people whose severe illness or injuries interfere with nutrition.*
- *Can improve the health of expectant mothers and their babies.*
- *Compensate for nutritional deficiencies in the treatment of alcoholism and eating disorders, and in the elderly and convalescents.*

DRAWBACKS
- *Not a substitute for sound nutrition from a varied diet.*
- *Several vitamins and minerals are hazardous in high doses.*
- *Wasteful and expensive if they provide more nutrients than the body can absorb.*

may need extra nutrients to promote their recovery.

Occasionally, healthy people also require supplements. During pregnancy, for example, doctors usually prescribe extra iron and folate, because most women have low stores of these nutrients. Many physicians also recommend extra calcium and a daily multivitamin pill. However, a pregnant woman should never take any supplements except those prescribed by her physician; excesses of some vitamins and minerals can be dangerous for both the mother and her developing baby.

Certain medications can interfere with the absorption of vitamins or minerals. Common offenders include blood pressure drugs, oral contraceptives, antibiotics, and over-the-counter painkillers and laxatives. People taking any of these medications may benefit from supplements if increasing dietary intake doesn't compensate for the nutritional drain. For example, doctors sometimes prescribe a potassium supplement when patients on diuretic or digitalis treatment can't get enough extra potassium from tomatoes, oranges, bananas, and other fruits and vegetables. Individuals on steroid medications may be advised to take calcium pills to help minimize the drugs' effects on the bones. If you are taking a medication, ask your doctor whether you need supplements.

Alcoholics usually need supplements to overcome their severe nutritional deficiencies. These have often resulted from an inadequate diet over a prolonged period of time and by overindulgence in alcohol, which interferes with the absorption of many nutrients. The latter problem may be compounded by liver disorders related to ALCOHOL USE.

When taken in high doses, vitamins and minerals assume pharmacologic properties and may be prescribed as drugs. High doses of niacin, for instance, may lower blood cholesterol, and vitamin E may be prescribed as an alternative to low-dose aspirin to protect against a heart attack.

COMMON MYTHS

Most theories about the benefits of megavitamin supplements haven't stood up to scientific scrutiny. Contrary to media reports, megadose vi-tamins have no proven value in treating schizophrenia, HYPERACTIVITY, and other brain or neurological disorders. Efforts to change criminal behavior with megavitamins have not been successful. And although deficiencies of vitamins B_6 and B_{12} can lead to depression and other mental disorders, B-complex supplements sold as "stress vitamins" do not help people cope with emotional tension.

While ANTIOXIDANTS such as beta carotene and vitamins A, C, and E have been associated with a reduced risk of cancer and other diseases, the evidence to date indicates that they have this effect only when consumed in foods—not as supplements.

Although smoking interferes with vitamin C metabolism, taking vitamin C supplements seems only to hasten the excretion of nicotine and thus increases the urge to smoke.

DANGEROUS DOSES

Taking high doses of certain vitamins and minerals can be harmful. A recent study involving healthy men found that about 200mg of vitamin C a day was an optimal amount. This is well above the 40mg RNI, but it is still a fraction of the megadoses often touted—without scientific proof—as preventing colds, cancer, and a host of other ailments. Many people mistakenly believe that even if high doses don't fulfill such promises, at least they're not harmful. In reality, vitamin C doses above 1,000mg a day can increase the risk of kidney stones and cause bladder irritation. In addition, about 10 percent of the population is genetically predisposed to conserve iron, a condition known as hemochromatosis. High doses of vitamin C increase iron absorption and can lead to iron overload in these susceptible people.

In high doses vitamin A causes liver damage, skin problems, fatigue, and other symptoms; taken before and during pregnancy, it can cause serious birth defects. High doses of vitamin D can result in calcium deposits in the heart and blood vessels; they also upset calcium metabolism and can lead to bone loss. Taken over an extended period of time, very large amounts of both vitamins can be fatal. Excessive zinc and several trace minerals have effects ranging from nausea and diarrhea to death if taken in doses that allow buildup in body tissues.

RISKY OR WORTHLESS

Although many supplements sold in health-food stores are promoted as having special health benefits, they are not subjected to the rigorous testing required for drugs. Most of these are of dubious benefit, and a few are even deadly. Ephedra, or ma huang, a herbal preparation marketed as a stimulant and weight-loss aid, has caused several deaths, even among people using it as directed. Millions of Americans take melatonin, a hormonal preparation that is touted as a remedy for insomnia and jet lag, and is said to delay the ravages of aging. The evidence for a positive risk-benefit ratio is so weak that the Canadian government does not allow the sale of melatonin supplements. Fish oil supplements contain high levels of cholesterol, as well as vitamins A, D, and K, which can accumulate to toxic levels when high doses are taken for a long time. Amino acid supplements have no proven dietary value and can lead to nutritional imbalances. Some may contain tyramine, which interacts with monoamine oxidase (MAO) inhibitor drugs, prescribed for depression.

URINARY TRACT INFECTIONS

CONSUME PLENTY OF

- *Nonalcoholic and caffeine-free fluids to flush out the urinary system.*
- *Cranberry juice and blueberries to acidify the urine.*
- *Citrus fruits and fresh fruits and vegetables for vitamin C.*
- *High-calcium foods and low-fat dairy products to reduce bladder irritability.*

AVOID

- *Bladder irritants, such as coffee, tea, and alcoholic beverages.*

Also known as cystitis, most urinary tract infections (UTIs) affect the bladder, but some may involve the kidneys, the ureters (the tubes that carry urine to the bladder), and the urethra (the tube through which urine exits the body). The most common symptom is an urgent need to urinate, even when the bladder is not full. Urination may

PREVENTIVE TACTICS

Hygiene measures can help women avoid recurrent UTIs; many doctors recommend the following.

- Wear loose-fitting white cotton underwear and panty hose that have cotton crotches.

- Avoid douching and using vaginal deodorants, which can cause bladder irritation.

- If you use a diaphragm, ask your doctor to check the size; one that is even slightly too large can irritate the urethra and bladder.

- Urinate and drink a glass of water before sexual intercourse and urinate within an hour afterward to flush out the urinary tract.

- After a bowel movement, wipe from the front to the back to reduce the risk of carrying intestinal bacteria to the urethra.

be accompanied by pain or burning and, in severe cases, small amounts of blood. There may also be a low-grade fever and an ache in the lower back.

Most urinary infections are caused by *E. coli* bacteria, organisms that live in the intestinal tract but that can travel to the bladder. Chlamydia, a sexually transmitted organism, is another cause of UTIs. Women are more vulnerable to urinary infections because the female urethra is shorter than that of males, and its location provides a convenient entryway for bacteria. Many women develop so-called honeymoon cystitis, inflammation caused by sexual activity or an oversize diaphragm.

ROLE OF DIET

Antibiotics are needed to cure bacterial urinary infections, but dietary approaches can speed healing and help prevent recurrences. Doctors advise drinking at least eight glasses a day of fluids to increase the flow of urine and to flush out infectious material. Avoid coffee, tea, colas, and alcoholic drinks, however; these increase bladder irritation. Naturopaths recommend drinking bearberry or celery seed herbal teas, which may be natural diuretics with anti-inflammatory properties.

Cranberry juice is a favorite home remedy, and one that is supported by research. Cranberries (and blueberries) contain a substance that speeds the elimination of bacteria by preventing them from sticking to the bladder wall. Most commercial cranberry juice is too diluted and overly sweetened, however, to be of much help. Health-food stores sell pure unsweetened cranberry juice, which can be made less tart by mixing it with apple juice. You can also use a juicer to create your own cranberry-apple juice.

Vitamin C helps strengthen the immune system, fight infection, and acidify the urine. And calcium may help reduce bladder irritability.

Case Study

After suffering three bouts of cystitis in less than a year, Jennifer, a 29-year-old loan officer, was referred to a specialist. Various tests failed to find any urinary tract abnormalities, but the urologist discovered a number of lifestyle factors that can contribute to recurrent bladder infections. Jennifer had been fitted with a diaphragm that was too large; she also used superabsorbent tampons as well as a vaginal deodorant.

For starters, the urologist suggested another method of birth control. He also recommended using pads instead of tampons and forgoing the deodorant, explaining that a daily shower was all she really needed. Finally, he suggested drinking 6 ounces of natural cranberry juice sweetened with an equal part of apple juice every morning and evening. Six months after making these changes, Jennifer was happy to report that she had not experienced any further symptoms of cystitis.

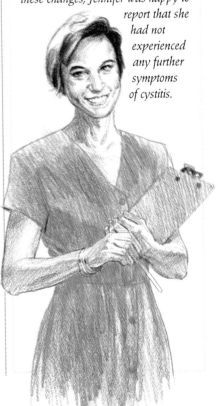

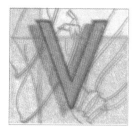

VAGINITIS

EAT PLENTY OF
- Dairy products, eggs, green and yellow vegetables, yellow and orange fruits, and fish for vitamins A and D.
- Fortified grains and cereals, poultry and seafood, bananas, dark green leafy vegetables, nuts, and seeds for B vitamins.
- Shellfish, beans, and legumes for magnesium and zinc.

CUT DOWN ON
- Foods high in refined sugar.

AVOID
- Fad diets for yeast hypersensitivity.
- Tight-fitting clothing.
- Irritating soaps and hygiene products.

If the acid-alkaline balance of the vagina is upset, yeasts and other microorganisms that are normally held in check by beneficial bacteria may proliferate. The result is vaginitis, a condition marked by itching, irritation, and inflammation. The usual causes are various species of yeast, most commonly *Candida albicans,* the protozoal organism *Trichomonas vaginalis,* and the bacterium *Gardnerella vaginalis,* which grows in oxygen-free conditions. Yeast infections can be identified by a cheesy discharge (unlike bacterial and protozoal infections, which are usually signaled by characteristic odors). In addition to itching and burning, symptoms may include an abnormal discharge, chafing, painful intercourse, and perhaps an urge to urinate more frequently than usual. However, some infections, such as chlamydiosis or trichomoniasis, may be present for years without symptoms.

Among the various conditions that may lead to vaginitis are lowered resistance due to fatigue, poor diet, or an infection elsewhere. Douching can upset the acid-alkaline balance, as can oral contraceptives. Hormonal changes that are brought about by pregnancy, diabetes, or menopause also increase vulnerability to vaginitis.

High blood sugar levels promote the growth of yeasts and other organisms, which is why diabetic women often develop vaginitis. Undiagnosed diabetes should be considered if a woman suffers unexplained bouts of vaginitis.

Women are particularly vulnerable to vaginitis when taking antibiotics for infections in other parts of the body. Certain antibiotics have side effects, including diarrhea and the overgrowth of natural yeasts, which can spread infecting organisms to the vagina. In menopausal women, low estrogen levels cause the vaginal walls to become thin, dry, and susceptible to abrasions that allow germs to enter.

DRUG TREATMENT
Doctors typically prescribe antifungal creams or pills to treat yeast infections; bacterial infections can usually be eradicated with antibiotics. While sexual partners often require treatment to prevent reinfection with bacteria or trichomonas, yeast infections may recur. Women taking certain antifungal pills should avoid alcohol; an interaction can cause a sudden rise in blood pressure.

Some topical antifungal medications are now available without a prescription. If you know the symptoms of yeast infection and your doctor agrees, you can try self-treatment. Follow the directions exactly; if you stop using the medication too soon, symptoms may recur and the yeast could become resistant to treatment. See a doctor if over-the-counter medication doesn't relieve symptoms within a day or two.

Menopausal women often find that vaginitis clears up after they begin estrogen replacement therapy. Using a vaginal lubricant during sexual intercourse protects tissues from abrasion and reduces the risk of infection.

HYGIENIC MEASURES
Changing the form of contraception may reduce the risk of vaginitis. Oral contraceptives change the vagina's acid-alkaline balance, which can foster the growth of yeasts and bacteria.

Women should avoid tight-fitting clothing that allows heat and moisture to build up in the vaginal area, encouraging yeast and bacterial growth. They should wear white cotton underwear and panty hose with cotton crotches. After vigorous exercise or swimming, they should change into dry clothing.

Feminine hygiene sprays and douches can irritate the vaginal mucous membranes. Some women douche with vinegar, but most doctors advise against this, because vinegar can harbor organisms that colonize the vaginal tissues.

HEALTHY FOODS
Although a link between diet and vaginal infections has not been proved, many doctors advise patients with recurrent infections to cut down on sugary foods. Many women claim that eating a daily portion of yogurt with active cultures prevents vaginitis, and recent studies seem to support this.

It's also claimed that allicin, an antibiotic in garlic, helps to stop yeast infections by blocking growth of the organisms. The protective effect may be obtained by eating raw garlic or taking garlic pills, however there is no way of knowing how much allicin garlic pills actually contain.

Cranberry juice protects against URINARY TRACT INFECTIONS; drinking it may prevent bacterial vaginitis from spreading to the bladder.

Research has linked low levels of vitamin A, the B vitamins, magnesium, and zinc with recurrent vaginal infections. Vitamin A, in particular, is necessary to keep mucous membranes and skin healthy and resistant to infections. Green and deep yellow vegetables and deep yellow and orange fruits are high in vitamin A. The omega-3 fatty acids in fish oils may reduce inflammation due to vaginitis; two or three servings of fish a week provide ample omega-3 fatty acids. Fortified grains and cereals, poultry and seafood, dark green leafy vegetables, potatoes, bananas, nuts, and seeds all provide the B vitamins. Good levels of magnesium and zinc can be obtained from frequent helpings of shellfish, beans, and legumes.

FAD YEAST-FREE DIETS

Several books have promoted strict yeast-free diets as a cure for yeast infections. There is no evidence that these fad diets are of any value. On the contrary, candida lives in the mouth, skin, and intestines of most healthy people, and eliminating these organisms with diet or drugs can be harmful.

HELPFUL FOODS

Deep green and yellow vegetables for vitamin A to maintain healthy mucous membranes that are resistant to infection. Have at least one serving daily.

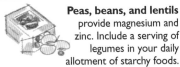

Peas, beans, and lentils provide magnesium and zinc. Include a serving of legumes in your daily allotment of starchy foods.

Yogurt and garlic are thought to protect against yeast infections. Eat low-fat yogurt daily; use garlic as a food flavoring or take in an odorless pill form daily.

VEGETABLES

BENEFITS
- *Many are rich in vitamins A, C, and E, folate and other B vitamins, and potassium and other minerals.*
- *High fiber content promotes regular bowel function.*
- *Rich in bioflavonoids and other chemical compounds that help prevent disease.*

DRAWBACKS
- *Eating large amounts may satisfy hunger without meeting energy needs.*
- *Goitrogens in cruciferous vegetables may interfere with thyroid function.*
- *Some are fairly common allergens.*

Because plants are capable of synthesizing energy from sunlight and air and combining it with minerals from the soil, they are the source of the nutrients essential to animal life.

Many of the plant foods that we call vegetables are, botanically speaking, fruits—these include green BEANS, cucumbers, eggplants, tomatoes, and even corn kernels.

Root vegetables, such as BEETS, carrots, parsnips, and turnips, are food storage organs and valuable sources of CARBOHYDRATES. Stems, such as celery and fennel, conduct nutrients between roots and leaves, and in some plants, such as potatoes and water chestnuts, underground stems have evolved into storehouses for starch. Vegetables with dark green leaves, including members of the cabbage family (such as broccoli, cauliflower, collard greens, kale, and mustard greens) and spinach, are rich in ANTIOXIDANTS, bioflavonoids, and the B vitamins, whether or not you eat the leaves. The leaves of all vegetables are factories for the production of high-energy sugars through photosynthesis. They are the most fragile parts of the plant, which is the reason they shrink more than other parts when cooked. The leaves of plants in the onion family have grown into fleshy bulbs that store carbohydrates and water to nourish the plant during its next year of growth. The flowers of some plants are also eaten; broccoli stems are eaten with their unopened flower buds and the flowers of zucchini are a delicacy.

HOW MUCH? OR HOW MANY?

The Food Guide Rainbow (see p.23) recommends 5 to 10 servings of fruits and vegetables daily. A serving is a half cup of raw or cooked vegetables, a cup of leafy salad vegetables, or a half cup of juice. Nutritionists recommend choosing from the cabbage family several times a week. In addition to antioxidants and bioflavonoids, these plants are teeming with the disease-fighting compounds known as phytochemicals and are rich in vitamins and minerals.

NUTRITIONAL VALUE

Green vegetables get their bright color from chlorophyll, the pigment that traps the energy from sunlight and makes it available for the production of sugars from water and carbon dioxide. Although chlorophyll is soluble only in fats, cooking vegetables in water liberates the enzyme chlorophyllase, which breaks chlorophyll down into water-soluble components. This has no nutritional consequence, but the green color of the vegetable is diminished. Some vitamins are also water-soluble, and are leached out into the cooking water.

Color is a useful guide to the vitamin content of vegetables. Plants produce vitamin C from sugars formed by photosynthesis in their leaves. The larger and darker the leaves are, the more

---

VEGETABLES GALORE. *Packed with vitamins, minerals, and phytochemicals that maintain health and help prevent cancer and other diseases, vegetables are the nutrition stars of the 1990s.*

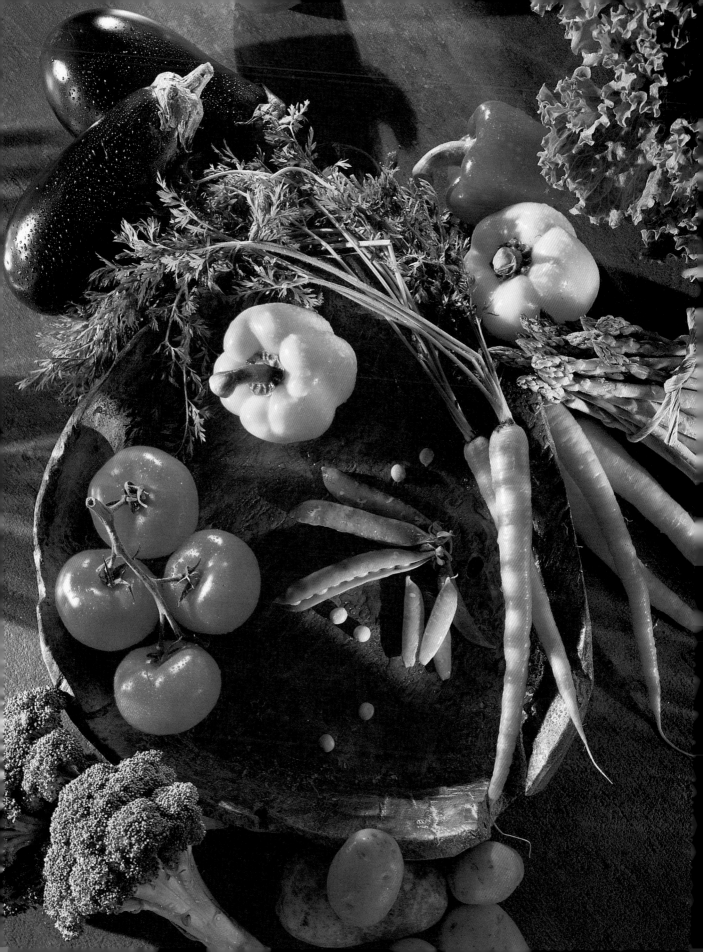

vitamin C and beta carotene they contain; the pale inner leaves of lettuce and cabbage, for instance, have only about 3 percent of the carotene found in the dark outer leaves. Unfortunately, outer leaves are often discarded because they are damaged or have been exposed to pollutants and pesticides.

Deep yellow, orange, or dark green vegetables derive their color from carotenoid pigments; these include beta carotene, an antioxidant that is converted to vitamin A in the intestinal wall. Because these pigments are stable in cooking and soluble in fat, the nutritional content is well preserved during baking or boiling.

Soluble and insoluble fiber in vegetables keeps bowel function regular and thereby reduces the colon's exposure to potentially toxic by-products of digestion. In some people, however, fiber can cause gas and bloating.

ANTICANCER FOODS

Cancer develops when mutant cells escape the body's protective immune system, allowing the growth of tumors made up of abnormal cells. Plants are also susceptible to cancer and have developed their own protective mechanisms. Vitamins A, C, and E are natural antioxidants that hinder cancer-causing cell damage by scavenging and inactivating free radicals, the unstable molecules that are released when the body uses oxygen. Some phytochemicals block the growth of blood vessels that feed tumors, others inactivate the enzyme systems that allow cancer cells to spread, and still others suppress the hormones that promote cancer growth. Studies have found that people who eat ample raw vegetables and fruits enjoy a reduced incidence of many cancers. By contrast, researchers have found that people who eat few vegetables are more prone to develop colon cancer.

Vegetables have a protective effect that is lacking in vitamin pills. Whole plants contain a balance of vitamins, minerals, fiber, phytochemicals, and as-yet-unidentified compounds. It is this blend that's important in blocking the effects of cancer-causing compounds.

PRESERVING NUTRIENTS

While vegetables provide starches, sugars, and proteins, their main contributions are vitamins, minerals, and fiber. Their nutrient content, color, and texture are affected by the method of preparation, the length of cooking time, and the volume of water used.

The yellow carotene pigments are not water soluble and are well preserved in cooking, but vitamin C and the B vitamins leach into the cooking liquid. Vitamin C is also quickly destroyed on exposure to oxygen. In addition, up to 20 percent of the vitamin C in a vegetable may be lost during each minute that it takes the water to heat from cold to boiling. This is because an enzyme that destroys vitamin C becomes more active as temperature rises; however, it stops its destructive action at the boiling point. For this reason, vegetables should be added to water that is already boiling. Steaming or cooking in a small amount of water retains more than twice the vitamin C that boiling does.

The yellow and orange carotenoid pigments are changed only by the high temperatures reached with pressure cooking. The brilliant green of chlorophyll in plant tissues is dulled, however, when heat causes chemical changes. The old-fashioned practice of adding a pinch of baking soda is not recommended—it produces a bright green color that breaks down the plant tissues, making the texture mushy and destroying many of the vitamins.

Color can be preserved by cutting vegetables into small, uniform pieces and cooking them rapidly; leafy vegetables needn't be cut. Using a large volume of water protects color, as it dilutes the color-destroying enzymes that seep out of the plant tissues, but it may leach out vitamins. Some cooks blanch such vegetables as beans and broccoli in boiling water for a minute or two, then plunge them into cold water to hold the color. This is satisfactory for vegetables that are served cold, but if they are served hot, they require rapid reheating, with further loss of nutrients.

STORAGE

Because harvested vegetables lose flavor, sweetness, and texture as they use their own food stores, the least amount of time stored, the better. Corn and peas can lose up to 40 percent of their sugar if kept at room temperature for just 6 hours after picking. Beans and stem vegetables, such as broccoli and asparagus, become tough.

Vegetables that originated in warm climates (such as beans, eggplants, peppers, okra, squash, and tomatoes) keep best at 50°F (10°C). Potatoes convert their starch to sugar below 40°F (4°C); keep them cool and out of the light to prevent the development of poisonous alkaloids. Most other vegetables keep best at 32°F (0°C). The salts and sugars in their sap prevent them from freezing until several degrees colder.

POSSIBLE HAZARDS

Most vegetables are safe to eat either raw or cooked. The exceptions are lima and kidney beans and other legumes, which contain toxic substances that are inactivated through cooking. Broccoli, kale, and other cruciferous vegetables harbor goitrogenic compounds that can interfere with iodine metabolism. Cooking inactivates these compounds, but eating large amounts of these vegetables raw may worsen a pre-existing thyroid condition.

Most vegetables do not provoke ALLERGIC REACTIONS, but some people react to members of the nightshade family such as eggplants and tomatoes. Corn is another common allergen.

VEGETARIAN DIETS: HEALTHY, ECONOMICAL, HUMANE

*A balanced vegetarian diet provides essential nutrients
while keeping weight down naturally. Also,
vegetarians have few ills linked to fat consumption.*

Until the most recent times, grains were the staple diet, while meat was a luxury reserved for the wealthy few. Today, in our affluent society with its huge surpluses of plant foods, we use grain to fatten stock animals. Critics contend that this is a wasteful use of resources, because it takes less grain to feed a person directly than it takes to fatten animals to feed that person.

On the whole, Canadians obtain about twice as much protein as is needed, and experts in medicine and nutrition warn that we are paying for our high consumption of meat and animal products with record rates of heart disease, stroke, certain cancers, and other disorders. A recent report by the Physicians Committee for Responsible Medicine, a group that advocates vegetarianism, claimed that Americans spend some $50 billion a year to treat illnesses related to a high-meat diet. However, many health experts have loudly criticized the report's findings as an overstatement.

Vegetarianism today has many adherents among people concerned with ecological issues, such as environmental pollution and population growth, as well as those who have age-old religious and philosophical concerns.

HEALTH BENEFITS

Although there is no scientific proof that vegetarians necessarily live longer than meat eaters, as a group they clear-

---

BENEFITS

- *Vegetarians are less likely to be obese or have heart disease; they also have lower blood pressure and fewer intestinal problems than meat eaters.*
- *A vegetarian diet is an economical use of the earth's resources.*

DRAWBACKS

- *Strict vegetarian diets may lack some vital nutrients.*
- *Diets restricted to plants may not be adequate for children.*

---

ly enjoy certain health advantages. For example, obesity is rare among vegetarians, probably because their diet is bulky and filling, high in fiber, low in fat, and relatively low in calories. They also tend to have lower blood cholesterol levels than meat eaters. Studies show that a cholesterol-free plant-based diet that is also low in saturated fats can reduce the risk of atherosclerosis, heart disease, and STROKE.

Vegetarians have lower blood pressure than meat eaters do and are less likely to develop hypertension, possibly because they have lower body weight and their diet is high in potassium. Intestinal disorders, such as constipation and diverticulosis, are rare among people who consume a high-fiber plant-based diet.

Several other disorders—including osteoporosis, kidney stones, gallstones,

and adult-onset diabetes—afflict vegetarians less often, although heredity, exercise, and environment are contributing factors as well.

ENSURING BALANCE

The nutritional needs of vegetarians are the same as those of omnivores and can just as easily be met by following the Food Guide Rainbow (see p.23). Adjustments must be made in a few areas, however, to make up for the lack of animal sources of several nutrients, namely protein, calcium, zinc, iron, vitamins D and B_{12}, and riboflavin.

Vegetarians must combine grains, seeds, and legumes to obtain PROTEINS with all the essential amino acids. Adults can achieve their amino acid balance by eating different plant proteins at separate meals in the course of a day, but children should be given both types of protein at the same meal. The Recommended Nutrient Intake (RNI) for protein is based on a diet including foods of both animal and vegetable origin. The daily needs for strict vegetarians are increased by 25 percent. For example, a 150-pound vegan should eat 68g of plant protein to match the 54g from mixed sources needed by an omnivore or ovolacto-vegetarian (a vegetarian who includes dairy products and eggs in his diet). Soy products are useful, because soy is the only plant source of complete protein.

Lactovegetarians (vegetarians who supplement plant foods only with

COMPLEMENTARY PROTEINS

Combining plant foods to make a complete protein can be as simple as eating a legume (peanut butter) with a grain (whole-wheat bread). Alternatively, nuts and seeds can be combined with dairy products or grains. Examples of complete-protein combinations are:

- Rice and beans.
- Bean-vegetable chili served with tortillas.
- Baked beans and corn bread.
- Hummus (made with chickpeas and sesame seeds).
- Cheese rolled in chopped nuts.
- Breadsticks with sesame seeds.
- Multigrain bread made with sunflower seeds.
- Macaroni and cheese.
- Split-pea soup sprinkled with cheese and served with a whole-wheat roll.

dairy products), ovolactovegetarians, and pescatarians (they include fish, dairy products, and eggs in their diet) can easily obtain most of the essential minerals from their diet. Tofu, dark green vegetables, seeds, nuts, fortified cereals, and whole grains are rich sources of calcium, zinc, and riboflavin and other B vitamins. Dairy products, egg yolks, and fish supply vitamin B_{12}.

A vegetarian diet may not provide enough iron, because people absorb only a fourth as much nonheme iron, which comes from plants, as the heme iron in meat, fish, and poultry. Every vegetarian meal should include foods high in vitamin C to promote iron absorption. In addition to citrus fruits, good sources include potatoes, cruciferous vegetables, peppers, melons, and strawberries.

Vitamin D is needed for calcium absorption; good dietary sources are egg yolks, fortified milk, and fatty fish. Exposure to sunlight enables the body to manufacture vitamin D.

It is more difficult for vegans and fruitarians (who eat only raw and dried fruits, nuts, honey, olive oil, and, perhaps, grains and legumes) to consume enough calories for energy and to achieve nutritional balance without supplements. Large helpings of nut butters, dried fruits, and breads can help maintain weight. Calcium-fortified soy milk or orange juice can help ensure adequate intake of this mineral. Nutritionists recommend iron and vitamin B_{12} supplements.

CHILDREN'S NEEDS

Strict vegetarians should plan for pregnancy and nursing by modifying their diets and taking supplements as advised by their obstetricians.

Parents should consult a dietitian for advice about a child's nutrition. While a balanced ovolactovegetarian diet can easily meet the demands of infancy, as well as CHILDHOOD AND ADOLESCENT NUTRITION, strict vegetarian diets are not recommended for babies and young children. Restricted vegan diets can hamper growth and development; undernourished children risk lifelong ill-health from rickets, iron-deficiency anemia, and other disorders. Vegan parents should plan meals with the advice of a registered dietitian who has special understanding of the child's needs. A pediatrician should monitor the child's growth.

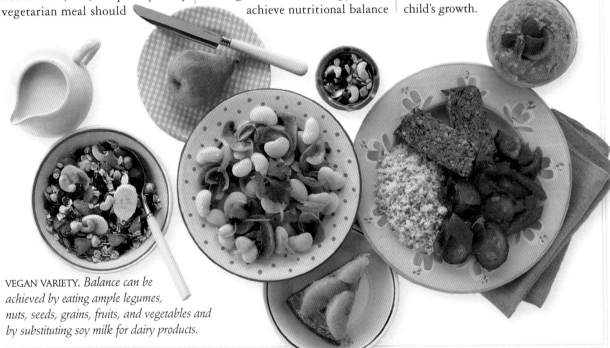

VEGAN VARIETY. *Balance can be achieved by eating ample legumes, nuts, seeds, grains, fruits, and vegetables and by substituting soy milk for dairy products.*

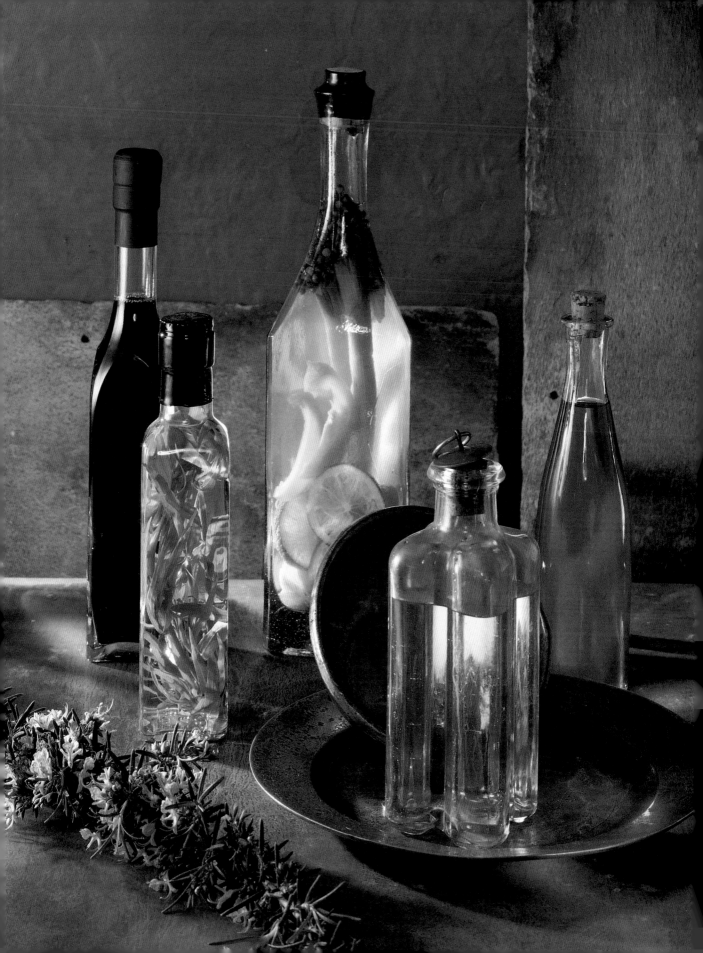

VERTIGO

EAT PLENTY OF
- *Low-fat high-fiber foods to prevent atherosclerosis.*

CUT DOWN ON
- *Salty and fatty foods.*

AVOID
- *Alcohol.*

Although many people use the terms *vertigo* and *dizziness* interchangeably, there are important differences between the two. Vertigo is characterized by an unpleasant illusion that you or your surroundings are spinning out of control, and it is often accompanied by severe nausea. In contrast, dizziness is less severe: light-headedness and an unsteady gait are the major features.

Vertigo usually stems from an imbalance of fluid in the inner ear, which affects one's sense of balance. It is a common complication of Ménière's disease, and it also occurs in older people with atherosclerosis.

Dizziness can originate in the ears too, but a more likely cause is hypotension, a temporary fall in the pressure of blood flowing to the brain. Other conditions that can cause dizziness include ANEMIA, fatigue, fever, heart disease, HYPOGLYCEMIA, various infections, STRESS, and motion sickness. Overindulgence in ALCOHOL can also produce dizziness.

ROLE OF DIET

People who suffer frequent attacks of vertigo are often advised to reduce their salt intake to help prevent a buildup of body fluids. A doctor may also prescribe a diuretic to reduce the body's fluid volume. To maintain good circulation and to prevent atherosclerosis, the diet should emphasize high-fiber, low-fat foods—fruits, vegetables, and legumes, grains, and other starches.

Other dietary approaches depend upon the underlying cause of the vertigo or dizziness. Those who experience attacks of dizziness when they are overly hungry may find that eating frequent small meals alleviates the problem. Although a low-salt diet may be indicated for vertigo, this is not the case for dizziness stemming from hypotension; some people actually need extra salt to maintain normal blood pressure. Attacks of dizziness can also be minimized simply by avoiding any abrupt movements of the head and by slowly assuming an upright position.

VINEGAR

BENEFITS
- *Basis for a low-calorie salad dressing.*
- *Can be used to preserve other foods.*

DRAWBACKS
- *May trigger an allergic reaction in people sensitive to molds.*

For centuries, vinegar was a by-product of wine and beer making; in fact, the name comes from the French word *vinaigre,* which means sour wine. Apple cider and wine remain the most popular basic ingredients, but almost any product that produces alcoholic fer-

---

THE PRICEY BALSAMICS

Rich, dark, and mild-flavored balsamic vinegar, which is produced from a type of red wine, originated in Modena, Italy. The most prized—and expensive—varieties are aged 15 to 50 years.

As a preserving liquid, vinegar has no equal: once sealed, it can last indefinitely. Any one of the balsamic, tarragon, citrus, wine or sherry vinegars pictured on p. 101 will enliven a salad.

---

mentation can be used to make vinegar, as evidenced by the dozens of varieties available today. Although vinegar probably lacks the healing power accorded to it by naturopaths, it provides a low-sodium, low-calorie flavoring.

All vinegars are 4 to 14 percent acetic acid. They are made in two stages. First, yeasts or other molds are added to turn the natural sugars in the basic ingredient into alcohol. Then, bacteria are introduced to convert the alcohol into acetic acid.

VARIETIES OF VINEGAR

Plain white (clear) distilled vinegar is the type used for making pickles and other condiments. It can be transformed into a flavored or gourmet vinegar simply by adding various herbs, spices, or fruits—for example, dill, tarragon, lemon balm, mint, garlic, green peppercorns, CHILIES, citrus, or RASPBERRIES. These and many other varieties are widely available, or you can make your own by adding fresh herbs or fruit to distilled, cider, or wine vinegars. Cover tightly and store in a dark cupboard. The acetic acid keeps the herbs or fruits from spoiling.

HEALTH BENEFITS

Herbalists and naturopaths often recommend various vinegars to treat arthritis, indigestion, and other ailments. Such claims have never been proved scientifically, but some arthritis sufferers insist that a tonic of cider vinegar and honey alleviates joint pain.

Vinegar is virtually devoid of calories, so it's an ideal alternative to fatty salad dressings. To reduce its acid bite, the vinegar can be mixed with orange juice or fruit syrup and a little oil.

A note of caution: People who are allergic to molds may react to vinegar as well as to foods preserved with it. Symptoms include a tingling or itching sensation around the mouth, and possibly hives.

VITAMINS

*Although the body can manufacture some vitamins,
most of them must come from the diet. A deficiency of any
of 13 essential vitamins can result in serious disease.*

For more than 2,000 years folk healers and physicians have known that eating certain foods prevents or cures diseases. In 400 BC, for example, Hippocrates found that eating liver cured night blindness. In 1747 James Lind, a British naval surgeon, advocated eating lemons and limes to prevent or cure scurvy, a disease rampant among sailors who subsisted on biscuits and salt pork on long voyages.

In 1912 Dr. Casimir Funk, a Polish biochemist, put forth the theory that foods contained essential chemical substances, which we now know as vitamins (see What's in a Name?, facing page). In 1913 vitamin A became the first vitamin to be identified by two separate American research teams.

To date, 13 vitamins essential to maintain health and prevent deficiency diseases have been discovered. Other vitaminlike substances—bioflavonoids, choline, carnitine, and taurine, among others—have also been identified. Some appear to be essential to health, but Recommended Nutrient Intakes (RNIs) for them have not been established. Researchers believe there are probably many more unknown vitamins, which is why they recommend eating a wide variety of foods to gain complete nutrition.

Only very small amounts—typically a few milligrams or even fractions of milligrams—of vitamins are needed to maintain good health. The Nutrition Research Division of Health

---

BENEFITS
- *Cure or prevent deficiency diseases, such as scurvy and rickets.*
- *Essential for energy conversion and many other metabolic processes.*
- *Antioxidant properties may help prevent cancer, heart disease, and other disorders.*

DRAWBACKS
- *High doses of some can be toxic.*

Canada has established RNIs for nine vitamins. The RNI is the amount needed to prevent deficiency diseases; however, it is not necessarily the optimum amount in terms of health. In general, eating a variety of foods in keeping with the Food Guide Rainbow (see p.23) will meet all the RNIs.

CLASSIFICATION

Vitamins are classified according to how they are absorbed and stored in the body. Vitamins A, D, E, and K are soluble only in fats, whereas vitamin C and the B vitamins are soluble in water. The body can store fat-soluble vitamins in the liver and fatty tissue. Since most excess water-soluble vitamins are excreted in the urine, they need to be consumed more often.

Provitamins are substances that the body can convert into vitamins; examples include beta carotene, a precursor of vitamin A, and a type of steroid in the skin that, after exposure

to the sun's ultraviolet rays, is used by the body to make vitamin D.

Antivitamins, or vitamin antagonists, are compounds in foods that can interfere with the action of real vitamins, to which they are chemically related. Though the body may recognize these substances as true vitamins and incorporate them into tissue, they are unable to carry out any functions.

FAT-SOLUBLE VITAMINS

These vitamins require the presence of fat in order to be absorbed from the intestinal tract. Thus, a person who has a fat-malabsorption disorder can develop deficiency symptoms even though the diet supplies adequate amounts of a vitamin. On the other hand, toxic amounts may build up if a person takes high-dose supplements or consumes an extraordinary amount of certain foods (for example, the huge amounts of polar bear and seal livers consumed by early Arctic explorers resulted in vitamin A toxicity).

Vitamin A. There are several forms of this vitamin—the preformed, or active, ones are retinol, retinoic acid, and retinyl esters. Beta carotene is a precursor form. Vitamin A, as the name *retinol* implies, is essential to normal vision and to prevent night blindness. But it is also necessary for normal cell division and growth, the development of bones and teeth, and for the health of skin, mucous membranes, and the epithelial tissue that lines the intestines, airways, and other organs. Its ANTIOXIDANT properties help prevent the cancer-causing cell damage of free radicals, unstable molecules that are released when the body uses oxygen. The body also needs Vitamin A to

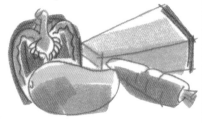

synthesize amino acids as well as thyroxine and other hormones.

Excessive vitamin A can cause toxicity, which can lead to death in extreme cases. A woman contemplating pregnancy should never take high-dose vitamin A supplements or isotretinoin (Accutane), a powerful acne drug derived from vitamin A. Because vitamin A is stored in the body, these should be stopped at least 3 months before attempting to conceive.

The amount of vitamin A may be listed in international units (I.U.) or retinal equivalents (R.E.). One R.E. is equal to 1mcg (microgram) of the retinol form of vitamin A, or 6mcg of beta carotene; 1 R.E. is equal to 3.5 I.U. from plant sources and about 10 I.U. of beta carotene.

Vitamin D. There are two forms of this vitamin: D_2, which comes from plants, and D_3, which the body synthesizes when the skin is exposed to ultraviolet (UV) rays from the sun.

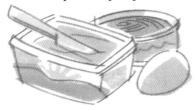

The body must have vitamin D in order to absorb calcium. It also promotes absorption of phosphorus and prevents the kidneys from excreting protein in the urine. Because of its role in mineral absorption, vitamin D promotes the growth of strong bones and teeth; deficiency causes rickets in children and osteomalacia in adults. Other deficiency symptoms include convulsions and muscle twitching.

Vitamin E. The tocopherols in vitamin E prevent the oxidation of vitamin A and fats, especially unsaturated fatty acids, in the intestinal tract and body tissues. They also help to maintain healthy red blood cells and muscle tissue, protect the lungs from pollutants, and regulate the synthesis of vitamin C and DNA. Recent studies indicate that when taken in high doses of 200 to 400mg a day, vitamin E may protect against heart attacks, stroke, and some aspects of aging. Unlike other fat-soluble vitamins, tocopherols do not accumulate to toxic levels in the body; instead, any excess is excreted in the stools.

Vitamin K. The liver requires vitamin K to manufacture blood proteins (Factors II, VII, IX, and X) that are es-

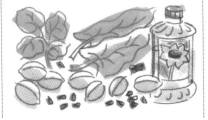

sential for blood clotting. Intestinal bacteria make half the needed vitamin K; the rest comes from the diet.

Deficiency is characterized by excessive bleeding from even minor cuts. Some newborn infants are especially vulnerable to vitamin K deficiency, because they lack the intestinal bacteria needed to make it.

WATER-SOLUBLE VITAMINS

As water-soluble vitamins, the B vitamins and vitamin C are more easily absorbed than the fat-soluble vitamins are, because there is always fluid in the intestines. At the same time, deficiencies may develop more quickly because the body stores water-soluble vitamins in only small amounts.

Biotin. Closely related to folate, pantothenic acid, and vitamin B_{12}, biotin is essential for the proper metabolism of carbohydrates, especially glucose, as well as proteins and fats. Some biotin is made by intestinal bacteria; it is also found in many foods. Deficiency occurs mostly in infants; in adults, it can be induced by eating lots of raw egg whites, which contain avidin, a substance that binds with biotin.

Folate. Also referred to as folic acid or folacin, this B vitamin is converted into enzymes that the body needs to

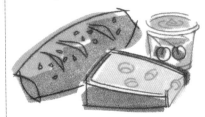

make DNA, RNA, and red blood cells, and to carry out other important metabolic functions. During pregnancy, folate helps prevent neurological defects, particularly a malformed spinal column, in the developing fetus. Recent research indicates that mild folate deficiency is common, especially among infants, adolescents, and pregnant women. Alcohol and oral

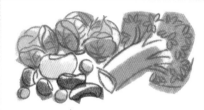

contraceptives interfere with absorption, increasing the risk of deficiency.

Niacin. Also known as vitamin B_3, nicotinic acid, and nicotinamide, niacin is important in energy metabolism, normal growth, and the synthesis of fatty acids, DNA, and protein. Mild niacin deficiency causes mouth sores and diarrhea; if unchecked, it can lead to pellagra, a disease characterized by chronic diarrhea, dermatitis, dementia, and if untreated, death.

When consumed in high doses (1,000mg or more per day), niacin may lower blood cholesterol levels. But such high doses should be taken only under careful medical supervi-

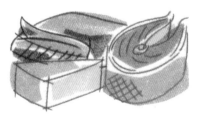

sion, with frequent blood checks for liver damage and high blood sugar.

Pantothenic acid. As implied by its name, which comes from the Greek term for widespread, pantothenic acid is found in almost all plant and animal foods; it is also manufactured by intestinal bacteria. Deficiency is unknown except in medical experiments.

Riboflavin. Essential for the release of energy, riboflavin is needed to metabolize carbohydrates, proteins, and fats. It is also necessary to utilize niacin and vitamin B_6, and it may play a role in the production of corticosteroid hormones. Riboflavin deficiency does not cause any specific diseases, but it can contribute to other B vitamin deficiency disorders.

Thiamine. Also known as vitamin

B_1, thiamine is instrumental in turning carbohydrates, proteins, and fats into energy; it is also needed to convert glucose into fatty acids. Still other important functions include promotion of normal nerve function, muscle tone, appetite, and digestion. A mild deficiency causes fatigue, listlessness, irritability, mood swings, numbness in the legs, digestive problems, and retarded growth in children. Severe deficiency leads to beriberi, a disease that now occurs mostly in alcoholics.

Vitamin B_6. Made up of three interchangeable and related compounds (pyridoxine, pyridoxamine, and pyridoxal), vitamin B_6 is a coenzyme that is essential for protein metabolism. It is needed to release energy in forms that the cells can use, and it is instrumental in the functioning of the nervous and immune systems and the manufacture of red blood cells. Deficiency is noted by oily, scaling skin, especially around the eyes, nose, and mouth; weight loss; muscle weakness; a smooth, red tongue; irritability; and depression. High-dose supplements can cause drowsiness and a loss of sensation in the fingers and legs.

Vitamin B_{12}. Like other B vitamins, B_{12} functions as a coenzyme with many roles. It is essential for the growth and division of cells, as well as for making red blood cells, genetic material, and myelin, the fatty sheath that surrounds nerve fibers. A deficiency can cause pernicious anemia, neurologic symptoms, and weakness.

The majority of cases of vitamin B_{12} deficiency in Canada is not due to

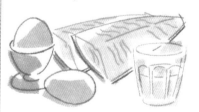

a poor diet; instead, it is almost always caused by an inability to absorb the vi-

tamin from the intestinal tract due to a lack of intrinsic factor. The stomach's production of intrinsic factor declines with age. Many intestinal disorders also result in inadequate intrinsic factor. In such cases, B_{12} must be injected; oral forms will not be absorbed.

Vitamin C. Also called ascorbic acid, vitamin C is necessary to make and maintain collagen, the connective tissue that holds body cells together. It promotes healing of wounds and burns, helps to build teeth and bones,

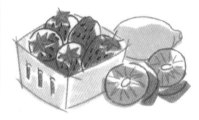

and strengthens the walls of capillaries and other blood vessels. Vitamin C increases iron absorption and is instrumental in the metabolism of folate, protein, and fats. In addition, it helps prevent atherosclerosis.

Vitamin C has not been proved to prevent colds, but deficiency does increase the risk of infection. More obvious deficiency symptoms are fatigue, joint pain, sore and bleeding gums, easy bruising, weakened bones that fracture easily, and slow healing of wounds. As these symptoms worsen into scurvy, gum ulcers form, the teeth loosen, and hemorrhages can develop.

A recent report found that 200mg a day may be closer to an optimal dose than the current RNI of 40mg. But many people persist in taking higher doses. Doctors warn that even a 200mg daily supplement can cause serious problems for anyone with a genetic tendency to store excessive iron. Very high doses (8g or more a day) can cause diarrhea, kidney and bladder stones, destruction of red blood cells, and loss of bone minerals.

VITAMIN	BEST FOOD SOURCES	ROLE IN HEALTH
FAT-SOLUBLE VITAMINS		
Vitamin A (from retinols in animal products or beta carotene in plant foods)	**Retinols:** Liver, salmon and other cold-water fish, egg yolks, and fortified milk and dairy products. **Beta carotene:** Orange and yellow fruits and vegetables, such as carrots, squash, and cantaloupes; leafy green vegetables.	Prevents night blindness; needed for growth and cell development; maintains healthy skin, hair, and nails, as well as gums, glands, bones, and teeth; may help prevent lung cancer.
Vitamin D (calciterol)	Fortified milk and butter; egg yolks; fatty fish; fish-liver oils. (Also made by the body when exposed to the sun.)	Necessary for calcium absorption; helps build and maintain strong bones and teeth.
Vitamin E (tocopherols)	Eggs, vegetable oils, margarine, and mayonnaise; nuts and seeds; fortified cereals; green leafy vegetables.	Protects fatty acids; maintains muscles and red blood cells; important antioxidant.
Vitamin K	Spinach, cabbage, and other green leafy vegetables; pork, liver, and green tea.	Essential for proper blood clotting.
WATER-SOLUBLE VITAMINS		
Biotin	Egg yolks, soybeans, cereals, and yeast.	Energy metabolism.
Folate (folic acid, folacin)	Liver; yeast; broccoli and other cruciferous vegetables; avocados; legumes; many raw vegetables.	Needed to make DNA, RNA, and red blood cells, and to synthesize certain amino acids.
Niacin (vitamin B_3, nicotinic acid, nicotinamide)	Lean meats, poultry, and seafood; milk; eggs; legumes; fortified breads and cereals.	Needed to metabolize energy; promotes normal growth. Large doses lower cholesterol.
Pantothenic acid (vitamin B_5)	Almost all foods.	Aids in energy metabolism; normalizing blood sugar levels; and synthesizing antibodies, cholesterol, hemoglobin, and some hormones.
Riboflavin (vitamin B_2)	Fortified cereals and grains; lean meat and poultry; milk and other dairy products; raw mushrooms.	Essential for energy metabolism; aids adrenal function.
Thiamine (vitamin B_1)	Pork; legumes; nuts and seeds; fortified cereals; and grains.	Energy metabolism; helps maintain normal digestion, appetite, and proper nerve function.
Vitamin B_6 (pyridoxine, pyridoxamine, pyridoxal)	Meat, fish, and poultry; grains and cereals; green leafy vegetables, potatoes, and soybeans.	Promotes protein metabolism; metabolism of carbohydrates and release of energy; proper nerve function; synthesis of red blood cells.
Vitamin B_{12} (cobalamins)	All animal products.	Needed to make red blood cells, DNA, RNA, and myelin (for nerve fibers).
Vitamin C (ascorbic acid)	Citrus fruits and juices; melons, berries, and other fruits; peppers, broccoli, potatoes; and many other fruits and vegetables.	Strengthens blood vessel walls; promotes wound healing; promotes iron absorption; helps control blood cholesterol and prevent atherosclerosis.

RECOMMENDED NUTRIENT INTAKES* (FOR ADULTS OVER 24)		SYMPTOMS OF DEFICIENCY	SYMPTOMS OF EXCESS
MALES	FEMALES		
1,000mcg R.E.	800mcg R.E.	Night blindness; stunted growth in children; dry skin and eyes; increased susceptibility to infection.	Headaches and blurred vision; fatigue; bone and joint pain; appetite loss and diarrhea; dry, cracked skin, rashes, and itchiness; hair loss. Can cause birth defects if taken in high doses before and during early pregnancy.
2.5mcg	2.5mcg	Weak bones, leading to rickets in children and osteomalacia in adults.	Headaches, loss of appetite, diarrhea, and possible calcium deposits in heart, blood vessels, and kidneys.
9mg	6mg	Unknown in humans.	Excessive bleeding, especially when taken with aspirin and other anticlotting drugs.
80mcg†	65mcg†	Excessive bleeding; easy bruising.	May interfere with anticlotting drugs; possible jaundice.
30–100mcg†	30–100mcg†	Scaly skin; hair loss; depression; elevated blood cholesterol levels.	Apparently none.
230mcg	185mcg	Abnormal red blood cells and impaired cell division; anemia; weight loss and intestinal upsets; deficiency may cause birth defects.	May inhibit absorption of phenytoin, causing seizures in epileptics taking this drug; large doses may inhibit zinc absorption.
19mg	14mg	Diarrhea and mouth sores; pellagra (in extreme cases).	Hot flashes; liver damage; elevated blood sugar and uric acid.
4–7mg†	4–7mg†	Unknown except in medical experiments; then fatigue, low blood sugar, numbness, digestive problems, and lowered immunity.	Very high doses may cause diarrhea and edema.
1.4mg	1mg	Vision problems and light sensitivity; mouth and nose sores; swallowing problems.	Generally none, but may interfere with cancer chemotherapy.
1.1mg	0.8mg	Depression and mood swings; loss of appetite and nausea; muscle cramps. In extreme cases, muscle wasting and beriberi.	Deficiency of other B vitamins.
2mg†	1.6mg†	Depression and confusion; itchy, scaling skin; smooth, red tongue; weight loss.	Sensory nerve deterioration.
1mcg	1mcg	Pernicious anemia; nerve problems and weakness; smooth or sore tongue.	Apparently none.
40mg	40mg	Loose teeth and bleeding gums; bruises; loss of appetite; dry skin; poor healing. In extreme cases, scurvy and internal hemorrhages.	Diarrhea; kidney stones; urinary-tract irritation; iron buildup; bone loss.

* Based on the Nutrition Research Division of Health Canada Recommended Nutrient Intakes (RNIs).

† No RNI has been established; this range is estimated to be safe and adequate.

GLOSSARY

*The following are important terms that do not
appear as separate entries in the book.*

ACUTE. Describes a condition that comes on quickly, produces marked symptoms, and rapidly reaches a peak.

ADIPOCYTE. A fat cell.

AFLATOXIN. A poison produced by molds that grow mainly on peanuts, cottonseed, and corn.

ALBUMIN. A protein found in most animal and many plant tissues that coagulates on heating.

ALKALOIDS. Nitrogen-containing compounds produced mainly by plants. Some (codeine, morphine, quinine) are used for medicinal purposes; others (nicotine, solanine in potatoes exposed to light) are poisonous.

ALLERGEN. A substance foreign to the body that causes an allergic reaction (see *Anaphylaxis*).

AMINO ACIDS. Organic (carbon-containing) acids that the body links to make proteins. Nine amino acids are termed essential, because they must be provided in the diet; the body produces the remaining 11 as they are needed.

ANAPHYLAXIS. An extremely severe allergic reaction that can be fatal; it occurs after repeated exposure to an antigen.

ANTIBODIES. Circulating proteins (immunoglobulins) formed by the body to resist future invasion by specific microorganisms or foreign substances (see *Antigen*).

ANTICARCINOGENS. Compounds that are thought to counteract certain cancer-causing substances.

ANTIGEN. A foreign substance that stimulates the body to defend itself with an immune response.

ARRHYTHMIA. An irregularity in the normal heartbeat.

ARTERIOSCLEROSIS. The stiffening and hardening of the arterial walls.

ASPARTAME. An artificial sweetener that is 200 times sweeter than sugar.

BACTERIA. Single-celled microorganisms that are found in air, food, water, soil, and in other living creatures, including humans. "Friendly" bacteria prevent infections and synthesize certain vitamins; others cause disease.

BASAL METABOLIC RATE. The energy required by the human body to maintain vital processes per 24-hour period.

B-GROUP VITAMINS. Although not chemically related to one another, many of the B vitamins occur in the same foods, and most perform closely linked tasks within the body. B vitamins are known either by numbers or names, or both: B_1, thiamine; B_2, riboflavin; B_3, niacin; B_5, pantothenic acid; B_6, pyridoxine; B_{12}, cobalamin; biotin; and folate.

BIOTIN. One of the B vitamins.

BOTULISM. A serious, often fatal, form of food poisoning caused by *Clostridium botulinum*.

CALCIUM. The most plentiful mineral in the body; a major component of bones, teeth, and soft tissues. Calcium is needed for nerve and muscle function, blood clotting, and metabolism.

CALORIE. The basic unit of measurement for the energy value of food and the energy needs of the body. Because 1 calorie is minuscule, values are usually expressed as units of 1,000 calories, properly written as kilocalories (kcal), or simply calories.

CARCINOGEN. A substance that can cause cancer.

CARIES. A decay of tooth or bone.

CAROTENES. Yellow and red pigments that color yellow-orange fruits and vegetables and most dark green vegetables. They are among the antioxidants that protect against the effects of aging and disease. The human body converts one such pigment—beta carotene—into vitamin A.

CELLULOSE. One of the main ingredients of plant cell walls, this indigestible carbohydrate is an important source of insoluble fiber.

CHLORINE. A nonmetallic element that is a necessary component of body cells and fluids, such as hydrochloric acid; it is found in gastric juice and is important to digestion.

CHROMIUM. A trace mineral that ensures proper glucose metabolism.

CHRONIC. Describes a condition that develops slowly or lasts a long time.

COBALAMIN. One of the B vitamins, also known as B_{12}.

COENZYMES. Compounds that work with enzymes to promote biological processes. A coenzyme may be a vitamin, contain one, or be manufactured in the body from a vitamin.

COFACTORS. Nonprotein substances that must be present before certain enzymes can function.

COLLAGEN. The fibrous protein that helps hold cells and tissue together.

COMPLEMENTARY PROTEIN. Protein-containing plant foods that lack one or more of the essential amino acids but can be paired with another plant food to supply a complete protein.

COMPLETE PROTEIN. A protein that contains all the essential amino acids. It's found in single animal foods; it can be constructed by combining two or more complementary plant foods.

COMPLEX CARBOHYDRATES. Starches and fiber that have a more complicated chemical structure than simple carbohydrates (sugars).

CONGENITAL. Present at birth, or inborn.

COPPER. A trace mineral necessary for the production of red blood cells, connective tissue, and nerve fibers. It is a component of several enzymes.

DEOXYRIBONUCLEIC ACID (DNA). The basic genetic material of all cells; the "genetic blueprint" that causes characteristics to be passed on from one generation to the next.

DIURETIC. A drug that causes the body to excrete excess urine.

ELECTROLYTES. Substances that separate into ions that conduct electricity when fused or dissolved in fluids. In the human body, sodium, potassium, and chloride are electrolytes essential for nerve and muscle function and for maintaining the fluid balance as well as the acid-alkali balance of cells and tissues.

ENDORPHINS. Natural painkillers made by the brain, with effects similar to those of opium-based drugs, such as morphine.

ENZYMES. Protein molecules that are catalysts for many of the chemical reactions that take place in the body.

EPINEPHRINE. Also called adrenaline, an adrenal hormone that prepares the body to react to stressful situations.

ESCHERICHIA COLI. Bacteria that occur naturally in the intestines of humans and other animals; one of the common causes of diarrhea and urinary tract infections.

ESTROGEN. A female sex hormone produced in both sexes, but in much greater quantities in females.

FETAL ALCOHOL SYNDROME (FAS). A constellation of mental and physical defects caused in the fetus by the mother's consumption of alcohol.

FOLATE. One of the B vitamins, also known as folic acid.

FREE RADICALS. Waste products of oxygen metabolism that can damage cell components.

FRUCTOSE. A naturally occurring, simple (monosaccharide) fruit sugar.

GASTROESOPHAGEAL REFLUX. When the lower esophageal sphincter opens at inappropriate times, food mixed with stomach acid flows back (refluxes) into the esophagus, causing indigestion and heartburn.

GLUCOSE. A simple sugar (monosaccharide) that the body converts directly into energy; blood levels of glucose are regulated by several hormones, including insulin.

GLYCOGEN. A form of glucose stored in the liver and muscles, which is converted back into glucose when needed.

GRAM (G). A metric unit of weight; one gram is equal to 1,000mg. There are 28.4g to an ounce.

HEME IRON. Iron that is found in hemoglobin in animal foods; the body absorbs about four times as much heme iron as nonheme iron, which is found in plants.

HEMOGLOBIN. The iron-containing pigment in red blood cells that carries oxygen.

HIGH-DENSITY LIPOPROTEINS (HDLS). The smallest and "heaviest" lipoproteins, they retrieve cholesterol from the tissues and transport it to the liver, which uses it to make bile; called "good cholesterol," because high blood levels of HDLs do not increase the risk of a heart attack.

HISTAMINE. A key chemical in the body's immune defense. Released during allergic reactions, histamine causes swelling, itching, rash, sneezing, and other symptoms.

HORMONES. Chemicals secreted by the endocrine glands or tissue; they control the functions of all the body's organs and processes, including growth, development, and reproduction.

HYDROGENATION. The process for transforming an oil (unsaturated liquid fat) into a hard fat by incorporating hydrogen. Hydrogenated fat is similar to saturated fat and linked to an increased risk of heart disease.

INCOMPLETE PROTEINS. Proteins, usually from plant sources, that lack one or more essential amino acids.

INDOLES. Nitrogen compounds found in vegetables and believed to protect against certain cancers by accelerating the elimination of estrogen.

INSOLUBLE FIBER. Fiber, such as cellulose, that passes undigested through the digestive tract.

INSULIN. A hormone that regulates carbohydrate metabolism.

IODINE. A mineral that is essential for the formation of thyroid hormones.

IRON. A mineral that is essential for the manufacture of hemoglobin and the transport of oxygen.

ISOTHIOCYANATES. Plant chemicals that are believed to strengthen the body's defenses against certain cancers (see *Phytochemicals*).

KETONES. Potentially toxic wastes produced from the body's partial burning of fatty acids for fuel.

LACTASE. An enzyme needed for the digestion of lactose.

LACTOSE. The natural sugar in milk.

LACTOVEGETARIAN. A vegetarian who consumes dairy products but no eggs, poultry, fish, meats, or other animal products.

LECITHIN. A phospholipid constituent of cell membranes and lipoproteins; a natural emulsifier that helps stabilize cholesterol in the bile. Lecithin is not an essential nutrient, because it is synthesized by the liver.

LINOLEIC ACID. One of the omega-6 essential fatty acids.

LINOLENIC ACID. One of the omega-3 essential fatty acids.

LIPID. A fatty compound made of hydrogen, carbon, and oxygen. Lipids are insoluble in water. The chemical family includes fats, fatty acids, carotenoid pigments, cholesterol, oils, and waxes.

LIPOPROTEIN. A combination of a lipid and a protein that can transport cholesterol in the bloodstream. The main types are high density (HDL), low density (LDL), and very low density (VLDL).

LOW-DENSITY LIPOPROTEINS (LDLS). These abundant, so-called "bad" lipoproteins carry most of the circulating cholesterol; high levels are associated with atherosclerosis and heart disease.

LOWER ESOPHAGEAL SPHINCTER. A muscular ring at the base of the esophagus; it opens to let food pass into the stomach and closes to prevent acidic stomach contents from flowing back (see *Gastroesophageal Reflux*).

MACRONUTRIENTS. Nutrients the body requires in large amounts for energy—specifically, carbohydrates, proteins, and fats.

MAGNESIUM. A trace mineral that is needed for healthy bones, the transmission of nerve signals, protein and DNA synthesis, and the conversion of glycogen stores into energy.

METABOLISM. The body's physical and chemical processes, including derivation of energy from food, that are needed to maintain life.

MICROGRAM (MCG). A unit of weight equivalent to 1/1000 milligram.

MICRONUTRIENTS. Essential nutrients that the body needs in only trace or very small amounts.

MICROORGANISM. An organism, such as a bacterium or virus, too small to be seen with the naked eye.

MILLIGRAM (MG). 1/1000 gram.

MONOUNSATURATED FATS. Fats that have one carbon-carbon double bond. They tend to be liquid at room temperature and semisolid or solid under refrigeration. They may help protect against heart disease.

MUCOUS MEMBRANE. The moist lining of the mouth, stomach, and many other cavities. It secretes a protective barrier of mucus, which serves as a lubricant as well as a medium for carrying enzymes.

NEUROTRANSMITTERS. Chemicals released from nerve endings that relay messages from one cell to another.

NITRATES. Nitrogen-containing compounds that occur naturally in certain foods. Used as preservatives in some meat products, as fertilizers, and in vasodilator drugs.

NITRITES. Compounds that are produced in the body by the action of bacteria on nitrates; also used as meat preservatives.

NITROSAMINES. Compounds that are formed in the body through the reaction of nitrites with amines in foods; regarded as carcinogenic, although no definite link has been established between nitrosamines and cancer in humans.

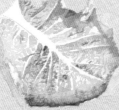

NONHEME IRON. Dietary iron obtained from plants; less well absorbed than iron from animal sources, although consumption with vitamin C (ascorbic acid) promotes absorption (see *Heme Iron*).

ONCOGENE. A gene for cancer; whether or not it is expressed (i.e., develops into cancer), and how fast, is affected by the diet.

OVOLACTOVEGETARIAN. A vegetarian who abstains from meat, poultry, and fish, but consumes eggs as well as milk and other dairy products.

OXALIC ACID. A potentially toxic chemical found in certain plants that inhibits the absorption of calcium, iron, zinc, and other minerals. Can promote the development of oxalate kidney stones.

OXIDATION. A chemical process in which food is burned with oxygen to release energy.

PANTOTHENIC ACID. One of the B vitamins.

PARENTERAL NUTRITION. Direct administration (through tubes inserted into the veins) of nutrient fluids into the bloodstream.

PASTEURIZATION. Heating of milk or other fluids to destroy microorganisms that might cause disease.

PECTIN. Soluble dietary fiber that regulates intestinal function and can help to lower blood cholesterol levels.

PERISTALSIS. Wavelike muscle contractions that help propel food and fluids through the digestive tract.

PHENYLKETONURIA (PKU). A genetic defect that prevents metabolism of the amino acid phenylalanine. People with PKU must follow a phenylalanine-free diet and avoid the artificial sweetener aspartame.

PHOSPHOLIPIDS. Waxy compounds, containing phosphoric acid, that are constituents of cell membranes.

PHOSPHORUS. A mineral needed for healthy bones and teeth, nerves, muscles, and for many bodily functions.

PHYTATES. Salts of phytic acid, found in grains and legumes, that hinder the absorption of minerals.

PHYTOCHEMICALS. Chemicals derived from plants; some have powerful effects, including both the prevention and the promotion of certain cancers, heart disease, and degenerative conditions linked to aging.

PHYTOESTROGENS. Plant chemicals with effects similar to those of the female hormone estrogen; found in yams, soybeans, and other legumes.

PLASMA. The clear yellow fluid that makes up about 55 percent of the blood and carries cells, platelets, and vital nutrients throughout the body.

PLATELETS. Disc-shaped cells, manufactured in the bone marrow, that are needed for blood coagulation.

POLYPHENOLS. Organic compounds, including tannins, that combine with iron and can hinder its absorption; found in a number of foods, tea, and red wines.

POLYPS. Small growths on mucous membranes; rarely malignant, although polyps in the lower bowel may become cancerous.

POLYUNSATURATED FAT. A fat containing a high percentage of fatty acids that lack hydrogen atoms and have two or more carbon-carbon double bonds. They tend to be liquid at room temperature.

POTASSIUM. A trace mineral that is needed to regulate fluid balance and many other functions (see *Electrolytes*).

PROSTAGLANDINS. Hormonelike chemicals involved in many body processes, including hypersensitivity (allergy) reactions, platelet aggregation (blood clotting), inflammation, pain sensitivity, and smooth muscle contraction.

PURINES. Compounds that form uric acid when metabolized; they are found in a number of foods, particularly high-protein foods, such as organ meats. Caffeine (in coffee and tea), theobromine (in chocolate), and theophylline (in tea) are related compounds. People prone to gout or kidney stones should avoid purines.

PYRIDOXINE. One of the B vitamins; more commonly called B6.

RECOMMENDED DIETARY INTAKE (RDI). Standards established by the World Health Organization (WHO).

RECOMMENDED NUTRIENT INTAKES (RNIs). Defined by Health Canada as the level of intakes of essential nutrients that will meet the needs of healthy people. The RNIs are expressed on a daily basis, but should be regarded as the average recommended intake over a period of about a week.

RIBOFLAVIN. One of the B vitamins.

RIBONUCLEIC ACID (RNA). A substance in every cell that enables the body to develop according to the information contained in the DNA.

SACCHARIDES. A term for sugars.

SALICYLATES. Compounds related to salicylic acid, which are used for making aspirin and other painkillers and as a preservative. Naturally occurring salicylates in fruits or vegetables may produce allergic reactions in people who are sensitive to aspirin.

SALMONELLA. A bacterium that is a frequent cause of food poisoning.

SATURATED FAT. A fat that contains the maximum number of hydrogen atoms. Found mostly in animal products, they tend to be solids at room temperature. They are linked to an increased risk of heart disease, certain cancers, and other diseases.

SELENIUM. An essential trace mineral with antioxidant properties.

SEROTONIN. A neurotransmitter that helps promote sleep and regulates many body processes, including pain perception and the secretion of pituitary hormones.

SODIUM. A trace mineral essential for maintenance of fluid balance; it combines with chloride to form table salt.

SOLUBLE FIBER. A dietary fiber that becomes sticky when wet and dissolves in water.

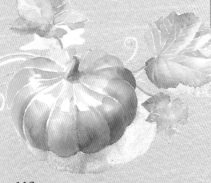

STAPHYLOCOCCUS. A family of bacteria that can cause disease, including skin infections and food poisoning.

STARCH. A complex carbohydrate that is the principal storage molecule of plants and the major source of carbohydrate and energy in our diet.

STEROIDS. A general class of compounds that includes hormones such as estrogen and testosterone. Synthetic steroids are used as anti-inflammatory drugs.

SUCROSE. A sugar composed of glucose and fructose. The sugar obtained from cane and beets; it's also present in honey, fruits, and vegetables.

SULFITES. Sulfur compounds that are used in food preservation and brewing. They may trigger asthma attacks.

SYNTHESIS. The process by which new compounds are created from components, such as new proteins assembled from amino acids derived from the proteins in food.

SYSTEMIC. Describing a condition or drug affecting the entire body.

TESTOSTERONE. A hormone that is produced in both sexes but primarily by the male testes.

THIAMINE. One of the B vitamins.

TOXIN. Any substance that is introduced into the body in a sufficient amount to cause an adverse effect.

TRACE NUTRIENTS. Nutrients, such as minerals, that are essential, though needed in very small amounts, to maintain health.

TRANS FATTY ACIDS. Fats that have been artificially hardened to remain solid at room temperature (see *Hydrogenation*).

TRICHINOSIS. A parasitic disease; it is caused by consuming *Trichinella* larvae in undercooked pork.

TRIGLYCERIDES. The most common form of dietary and body fat; high blood levels have been linked to heart disease.

TRYPTOPHAN. An essential amino acid found in many animal foods; a precursor of serotonin. Its use as a dietary supplement has been linked with serious illness, most likely due to contamination during the manufacturing process.

UREA. A waste product of the breakdown of protein, which is excreted by the kidneys.

URIC ACID. A nitrogen-containing waste product of protein metabolism. Buildup in the body causes gout.

VEGAN. A strict vegetarian who consumes no animal products.

VERY LOW DENSITY LIPOPROTEINS. A fat-carrying protein that transports mostly triglycerides in the blood.

VIRUS. Infectious, disease-causing particles that reproduce by invading and taking over living cells.

WATER-SOLUBLE VITAMINS. Vitamins that dissolve in water, specifically vitamin C and the B-group vitamins.

XANTHINES. Alkaloid compounds that occur in many plants, including coffee (caffeine), cocoa (caffeine, theobromine), tea (caffeine, theobromine, theophylline), and cola nuts (caffeine); related to *Purines*.

ZINC. A trace mineral that is essential for many processes, including metabolism, the healing of wounds, and normal growth.